MARY SHERIDAN'S
FROM BIRTH TO FIVE YEARS

Mary Sheridan's From Birth to Five Years: Children's developmental progress, based on the pioneering work of Mary Sheridan, is widely regarded as the go-to reference for health, education and social care professionals, or anyone concerned with the developmental progress of pre-school children.

In this new fourth edition, the text has been developed to further align it with current research and practices, and to support the wider group of professionals who are now required to take steps to promote children's development as part of their assessment and management plans. This book aims to provide the knowledge required for understanding children's developmental progress with age and within each developmental domain.

Features of this completely revised edition include:

- for students and tutors – information on theoretical aspects of development, with further reading suggestions;
- expanded sections on self-regulation of emotions and attention and attachment, temperament and the development of self;
- a new section on early literacy development.

To consolidate and expand on the practical and theoretical information across this book and its companion volume, *From Birth to Five Years: Practical developmental examination*, a new companion website is available at **www.routledge.com/cw/sharma**, which includes the following additional learning material:

- a timeline of the key developmental domains;
- introductions to theories of development, with links to further reading;

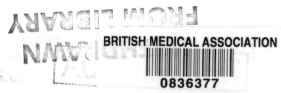

- further detail on topics signposted in the text;
- video clips demonstrating practical assessment skills.

Ajay Sharma is a Consultant Community Paediatrician at Guy's and St Thomas' NHS Foundation Trust, Southwark, London.

Helen Cockerill is a Consultant Speech and Language Therapist at the Evelina London Children's Hospital, Guy's and St Thomas' NHS Foundation Trust.

MARY SHERIDAN'S
FROM BIRTH TO FIVE YEARS

Children's developmental progress

Fourth Edition

Ajay Sharma and Helen Cockerill

Illustrations by Nobuo Okawa

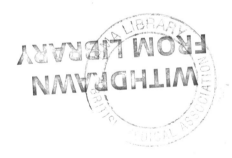

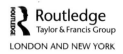
Routledge
Taylor & Francis Group

LONDON AND NEW YORK

First edition published 1973
by the NFER Publishing Company Ltd.

This edition published 2014
by Routledge
2 Park Square, Milton Park, Abingdon, Oxon, OX14 4RN

and by Routledge
711 Third Avenue, New York, NY 10017

Routledge is an imprint of the Taylor & Francis Group, an informa business

British Library Cataloguing in Publication Data
A catalogue record for this book is available from the British Library

Library of Congress Cataloging-in-Publication Data
Sharma, Ajay, author.
  Mary Sheridan's from birth to five years. Children's developmental
  progress / by Ajay Sharma and Helen Cockerill. — 4th edition.
    p. ; cm.
  title: From birth to five years. Children's developmental progress
  Preceded by: From birth to five years : children's developmental
  progress / Mary D. Sheridan. 3rd ed. / rev. and updated by Ajay Sharma
  and Helen Cockerill. 2008.
  Complemented by: From birth to five years. Practical developmental
  examination / by Ajay Sharma and Helen Cockerill. 2014.
  Includes bibliographical references and index.
  I. Cockerill, Helen, author. II. Sheridan, Mary D. (Mary Dorothy).
  From birth to five years. 2008. Preceded by (work): III. Sharma, Ajay.
  From birth to five years. Practical developmental examination.
  Complemented by (work): IV. Title. V. Title: From birth to five years.
  Children's developmental progress.
  [DNLM: 1. Child Development. 2. Child, Preschool. 3. Infant. WS 105]
  RJ131
  618.92—dc23   2013033534

ISBN13: 978-0-415-83353-0 (hbk)
ISBN13: 978-0-415-83354-7 (pbk)
ISBN13: 978-0-203-49456-1 (ebk)

Typeset in Univers by
Keystroke, Station Road, Codsall, Wolverhampton

Contents

A visual tour of the book

Key developmental milestones

The key *developmental milestones* for each *domain* are provided as boxed features, to consolidate the concepts explained in the main text and provide a quick reference for students and practitioners.

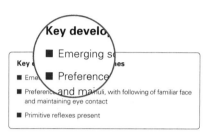

Illustrated charts

Charts of children's developmental progress are provided, organised by *domain*, and illustrations are provided to offer visual representations of the milestones being discussed.

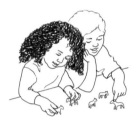

joins in make-believe play with other children

Links to website and companion volume

In this new edition of *From Birth to Five Years*, visual indicators have been added to the text to enable easy cross-referencing between this book and its new companion volume, *From Birth to Five Years: Practical developmental examination*, and the companion website that contains supplementary online material relevant to both books.

Whenever you see a boxed feature like this in the margin, look for the related section in the companion volume ('Hearing and Vision', in this example).

> ***From Birth to Five Years – Practical Developmental Examination***
>
> Hearing and Vision

Primitive and
protective reflexes
in infancy

Whenever you see a boxed feature like this in the margin, with the @ symbol, look for the related supplementary material on the companion website ('Primitive and protective reflexes in infancy', in this example).

Non-verbal cognitive
development

Whenever you see a boxed feature like this in the margin, with a 'play video' symbol, look for a related practical assessment skills instructional video on the companion website ('Non-verbal cognitive development', in this example).

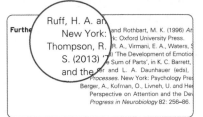

Further reading and references

Each chapter in Section 2 of the book concludes with a list of key scholarly books and articles, useful for practitioners to expand their knowledge of the theories and concepts covered, and helpful for students developing and researching essays and assignments. A full list of references is also included at the end of the book.

Glossary

Key terms are highlighted in *italic* within the text, and defined in a comprehensive glossary at the end of the book.

Introduction

Dr Mary D. Sheridan was a pioneer in UK developmental paediatrics in the 1960s. She created the concept of periodic developmental assessment of young children and stimulated the setting up of courses for community doctors and general practitioners. Her booklet 'Developmental Progress of Infants and Young Children', written in 1960, later became the first edition of *From Birth to Five Years* in 1973. The original edition was primarily concerned with describing developmental *norms* for the purposes of detecting and diagnosing disorders

Subsequent editions of *From Birth to Five Years*, in 1977 and 2008, continued to have Mary Sheridan's careful observations of children's developmental progress at the core of the work, but also widened the focus to encompass not only what children do, but also the process of development, based on the latest research.

Surveillance and monitoring of children's progress are clearly not the preserve of doctors. A range of professionals in health, education and social care are involved in the observation and assessment of children, and subsequent editions of *From Birth to Five Years* have provided concise and clear information to guide this process. The current edition, authored by a Community Paediatrician and a Speech and Language Therapist, aims to contribute to the core knowledge and skills of everyone who works with young children, and are involved therefore in improving health, educational and social outcomes.

Section 1 provides illustrated charts of children's developmental progress, organised into domains: posture and large movements; visual perceptual and fine motor; speech, language and communication; social behaviour and play; self-care and independence.

The charts for infants also include descriptions of hearing, vision and other senses. The content of the charts has been updated to reflect changes in our understanding of the processes underlying development: in particular, there is an increased emphasis on social communication, perception and *attention* control. Key developmental milestones are given for each age band. The division into domains is an artificial but pragmatic construct, designed to make information easily manageable. However, it is well recognised that domains overlap and integrate within the dynamic process of development.

Section 2 provides information on the sequence of development within each domain. These chapters also explore influences on the process of development, with some discussion of child- and context-related risks and protective factors. Additional information is given on key aspects of development that are not typically captured in domain-based developmental charts, including self-regulation, emotions and attention, and also attachment, temperament and the development of self. Early literacy development is given a new chapter in recognition of the importance of literacy readiness in influencing educational achievement after the age of 5. Each chapter provides guidance on strategies to support children's progress.

The primary purpose of this volume is to provide information rather than to be a checklist to assess an individual child's progress against a set of expected milestones. Development does not progress at the same rate in all children – there is broad variation in 'typical' ages of achieving milestones. Most children, however, follow a similar pattern or sequence of development. Reference is made in the text to developmental variation, particularly in relation to motor and language development.

Alongside this edition the authors have developed a companion volume: *From Birth to Five Years: Practical developmental examination*. This is aimed at providing practical guidance on evaluating children's developmental progress, usually in response to questions that have been raised by carers or other professionals. The purpose of developmental examination is to verify concerns, to elicit and categorise developmental function and any likely risk or impairment, provide support and guidance and arrange further assessment and/or investigations as required. *Practical developmental examination* also discusses risk and protective factors in greater depth.

Throughout the text signposts are given to further information provided on the companion website. This includes key developmental theories, and concepts such as joint attention, social cognition and bilingualism.

Finally, the website contains a timeline and linked video clips of children demonstrating a range of developmental skills across the domains, from birth to 5 years.

Illustrated charts of children's developmental progress

The newborn comes to this world with a rich repertoire of motor and perceptual skills acquired *in utero*. These skills enable the newborn to start a secure attachment and continuing reciprocal relationship with caregivers, and learn about them and the environment. Observing the neurodevelopmental status of the newborn provides a window into the health of the antenatal process, reassures parents and helps establish a basis for observing future progress.

THE NEWBORN BABY

During the first few days of life, there is a great variability in the behaviour of babies depending not only upon the baby's maturity and physical condition but also upon its state of alertness or drowsiness, hunger or satiation.

Alertness and responsiveness

- The first few days of a baby's life are usually composed of long periods of sleep interspersed with short periods when the baby is awake.

- The duration of wakefulness lengthens gradually and includes periods of fretfulness, crying and calmness.

- The responsiveness of the baby depends on the state of sleep or wakefulness (Brazelton and Nugent 1995).

Posture and large movements

- At birth, due to weak muscles, movements are mainly limited to arms and legs. The *muscle tone* is increased in the limbs and decreased in trunk and neck – when pulled to sitting, marked head lag is present and in a supported sitting position, the back is curved, and the head falls forward.

- Arms and legs are kept semi-flexed when lying on back (supine). However, babies born after breech presentation usually keep their legs extended.

- When the infant is held in ventral suspension, the head drops below the plane of the body, and the arms and legs are kept partly flexed.

- In prone position (on the abdomen), the head is promptly turned sideways. The buttocks are humped up, with the knees tucked under the abdomen. The arms are close to the chest with the elbows fully flexed.

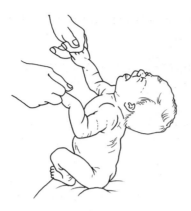
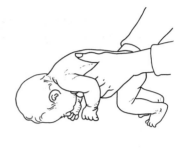

pulled to sit   *ventral suspension*

The primitive reflexes

Primitive and protective reflexes in infancy

Primitive reflexes are complex automatic movement patterns, generated by the lower brain (brainstem). They commence as early as 25th week gestation and are fully present at birth in term infants. They become more and more difficult to elicit over the coming months as cortical inhibition emerges and protective postural reactions begin to appear. Persistence and asymmetry of primitive reflexes may indicate an underlying neurological impairment.

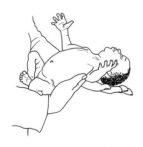

Moro reflex

■ The Moro reflex is the best known of all the primitive reflexes. It can be produced in several ways. The usual method is by sudden, slight (2.5 centimetres) dropping of the examiner's hand supporting the baby's head. The response consists of symmetrical wide abduction of the arms and opening of the hands. Within moments, the arms come together again, simulating an embrace. The reflex fades rapidly and is not normally present after 6 months of age.

■ Reflex rooting and sucking behaviour is apparent unless the baby has just been fed. Infants show nutritive sucking for feeding and non-nutritive sucking patterns (self-calming on fingers or dummies). Rooting fades by 6 months and involuntary sucking by 12 months.

■ Protective gag and cough reflexes are also present, and these persist throughout life.

■ Strong and symmetrical palmar grasp reflex is present but fades rapidly over the next 4 to 5 months.

■ Reflex standing and reflex walking are apparent during the early weeks of life if the feet are placed on a firm surface.

Hearing and vision

■ Babies are sensitive to light and sound at birth though visual responsiveness varies. From birth onwards, or within a few days, infants turn their eyes towards a large and diffuse source of light and close their eyes to sudden bright light. Infants show a preference for looking at faces or patterns. *Visual acuity* is poor at birth (20/200), rapidly reaching adult values of 20/20 by the end of first year. An object or face must be brought to a distance of 30 centimetres to obtain interest and fixation. Infants usually turn their eyes to slowly follow a face.

■ Infants can hear sounds in the last few months of pregnancy and show recognition of the mother's voice and of their native language soon after birth.

■ The startle reaction to sudden loud sounds is present. Eyes may be turned towards a nearby source of continued sound, such as a voiced 'ah-ah' or a bell. Momentary stilling to weaker, continuous sounds is also seen.

Touch, smell and taste

Babies are particularly sensitive to touch on the mouth, face, hands, soles and abdomen. Stroking, rubbing and skin-to-skin contact is the human equivalent to licking in other primates. There is evidence that skin-to-skin contact between the newborn and the mother in the immediate postpartum period may have positive effects on breastfeeding success and on maternal blood pressure and cortisol levels.

Newborns recognise the mother by her smell. They show a smile-like response (tongue protrusion, lip smacking, lip sucking) to sweetened solution – it also calms them and reduces their heart rate, but they purse their lips after being given a sour solution.

Social interaction

■ Within a few days of birth, infants establish interaction with their carers through eye contact, spontaneous or imitative facial gestures (protruding their tongue or pouting their mouth) and modulation of their sleep–wakefulness state. They show some recognition of their mother's smell and voice by becoming more relaxed, settled and happy.

■ Patterns of interaction and subtle indications of individuality shown by babies from birth onwards strengthen the emotional ties between infants and their carers.

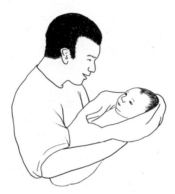

social interaction

Key developmental milestones

■ Emerging *social smile*

■ Preference for social stimuli, with following of familiar face and maintaining eye contact

■ Primitive reflexes present

■ Lying on back (supine), keeps head to one side. Moves arms and legs in large, jerky movements. At rest, keeps hands closed and thumbs turned in, but beginning to open hands from time to time. Fingers and toes fan out during extensor movements of limbs.

Posture and large movements

■ When cheek touched at corner of mouth, turns head to same side in attempt to suck finger (rooting reflex). Pulled to sit, head lags unless supported.

■ Held in supported sitting, head is vertical momentarily before falling forwards, and back is one complete curve.

Primitive and protective reflexes in infancy

■ In ventral suspension, holds head in line with body and hips are semi-extended.

■ Placed on abdomen (prone), head immediately turns to side; arms and legs flexed, elbows away from body, buttocks moderately high.

■ Held standing on hard surface, presses down feet, straightens body and usually makes a reflex forward 'walking' movement. Stimulation of dorsum of foot against table edge produces 'stepping' reflex.

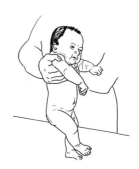

reflex 'walking' movement

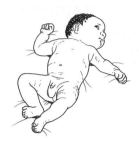

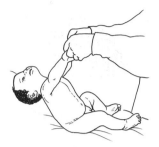

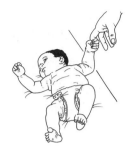

lying on back supine (showing asymmetric tonic neck reflex)

head lag on pulled to sit

grasps finger

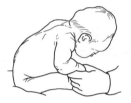

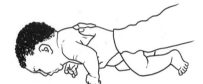

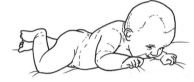

held sitting

ventral suspension

attempts to lift head in prone

Visual perceptual and fine motor

■ Pupils react to light. Turns head and eyes towards diffuse light source – stares at diffuse brightness of window, table lamp or lightly coloured blank wall.

■ Follows pencil light briefly with eyes, at a distance of 30 centimetres. Shuts eyes tightly when pencil light shone directly into them.

■ Gaze caught and held by dangling bright toy gently moved in line of vision at 15–25 centimetres, towards and away from face. From about 3 weeks, watches familiar nearby face when being fed or talked to with increasingly alert facial expression. Focuses and follows, with eyes, slow movements of face or object from side towards midline horizontally, with some accompanying head movement through quarter circle or more, before head falls back to side.

■ Defensive blink present by 6–8 weeks.

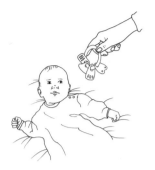

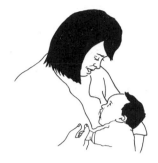

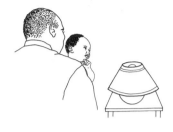

gazes at toy moved towards and away from face

regards familiar face when being fed

turns to diffuse light source

■ Startled by sudden noises, stiffens, quivers, blinks, screws up eyes, extends limbs, fans out fingers and toes and may cry.

■ Movements momentarily 'frozen' when small bell rung gently; may move eyes and head towards sound source, but cannot yet localise sound.

Hearing behaviour

■ Stops whimpering; and usually turns towards sound of nearby soothing human voice or loud and prolonged noise, e.g. vacuum cleaner, but not when screaming or feeding.

Speech, language and communication

■ Utters little *guttural noises* and vowel-like vocalisations when content.

■ Babies have a preference for social stimuli and will move arms and legs, and make active facial and pre-speech lip and tongue movements responsively to parent's or carer's talk from soon after birth.

■ Cries lustily when hungry or uncomfortable.

Note: babies with hearing impairment also cry and vocalise in this reflex fashion but when very severely impaired do not usually show startle reflex to sudden noise. Babies with severe visual impairment may also move eyes towards a sound-making instrument. Visual following and auditory response must, therefore, always be tested separately.

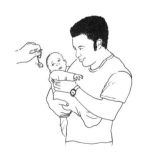

stops whimpering to listen to sudden noise

Social cognition:
Early interaction
patterns

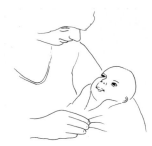

Eye contact and social smile

Social behaviour and play

■ Sleeps most of the time when not being fed or handled.

■ Expression still vague but becoming more alert, progressing to *social smile* and responsive vocalisations at about 5 or 6 weeks.

■ Eye-to-eye contact is deliberately maintained or terminated by the infant during social interaction.

■ Hands normally closed, but if opened, grasps finger when palm is touched.

■ Stops crying when picked up and spoken to. Turns to regard nearby speaker's face.

Self-care and independence

■ Sucks well.

■ Needs support to head when being carried, dressed and bathed.

■ Passive acceptance of bathing and dressing routines gradually gives way to emerging awareness and responsiveness.

AGE 3 MONTHS

Key developmental milestones

■ Head control in supported sitting

■ Visual following of face/toy, in a semi-circle

■ Visual hand regard in midline

■ Responsive vocalisation (proto-conversations)

Posture and large movements

■ Lying on back, prefers to lie with head in midline. Limbs more pliable. Movements smoother and more continuous. Waves arms symmetrically. Hands loosely open.

■ Brings hands together in midline over chest or chin. Kicks vigorously, legs alternating or occasionally together.

■ When pulled to sit, little or no head lag. Held sitting, back is straight except in lumbar region. Head held erect and steady in supported sitting (3–4 months).

■ In ventral suspension, head held well above line of body, hips and shoulders extended.

■ Needs support at shoulders when being bathed and dressed.

■ Lying on abdomen, lifts head and upper chest well up in midline, using forearms to support (1–4 months) and often actively scratches at surface with hands, with buttocks flat.

■ Held standing with feet on hard surface, sags at knees.

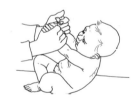

pulled to sit

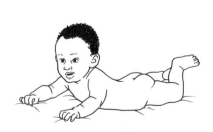

lifts head and shoulders in prone

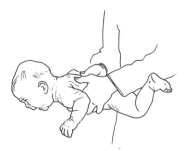

ventral suspension

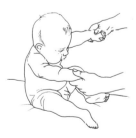

held sitting, with steady head

Visual perceptual and fine motor

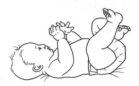

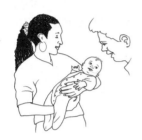

hand regard and finger play

turns to nearby voice

■ Visually very alert. Particularly preoccupied by nearby human face. Moves head deliberately to gaze attentively around. Follows adult's movements within available visual field.

■ Follows dangling toy at 15–25 centimetres from face through half circle horizontally from side to side and usually also vertically from chest to brow. Defensive blink is clearly shown.

■ Hand regard when lying supine – watches movement of own hands before face and engages in finger play, opening and closing hands and pressing palms of hands together.

■ Regards small still objects within 15–25 centimetres for more than a second or two, but seldom fixates continuously.

■ Eyes converge as dangling toy is moved towards face.

■ Reaches out to grasp with both hands by 16–18 weeks of age.

■ Holds rattle for a few moments when placed in hand, may move towards face – sometimes bashing chin – but seldom capable of regarding it at the same time until 16–18 weeks of age.

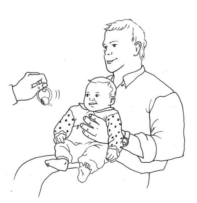

follows dangling toy

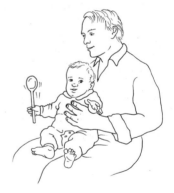

holds toy but cannot yet coordinate hands and eyes

Hearing behaviour

■ Turns eyes and/or head towards sound source, e.g. nearby voice; brows may wrinkle and eyes dilate.

■ May move head from side to side as if searching for sound source.

■ Quietens to sound of rattle or small bell rung gently out of sight.

■ Definite quieting or smiling to sound of familiar voice before being touched, but not when screaming.

Note: babies with severe hearing impairment may be obviously startled by carer's appearance beside cot.

■ Cries when uncomfortable or annoyed.

■ Often sucks or licks lips in response to sounds of preparation for feeding.

■ Shows excitement at sound of approaching voices, footsteps, running bathwater, etc.

■ Vocalises delightedly when spoken to or pleased; also when alone. Vocalisations are integrated with smiles, eye contact and hand gestures during turn-taking exchanges or 'proto-conversations'.

Speech, language and communication

■ Fixes eyes unblinkingly on parent's or carer's face when feeding, with contented purposeful gaze.

■ Eager anticipation of breast or bottle feed. Beginning to show reactions to familiar situations by smiling, cooing and excited movements.

■ Now definitely enjoys bathing and care routines. Responds with obvious pleasure to friendly handling, especially when accompanied by playful tickling, child-directed speech and singing.

Social behaviour and play

Child-directed speech

responds with pleasure to friendly handling

AGE 6 MONTHS

Key developmental milestones

■ Weight bearing on supported standing

■ Rolling from front to back

■ Primitive reflexes have abated and protective reflexes begin to appear

■ Reaches out with one hand to grasp (palmar), passes objects from hand to hand

■ Monosyllabic *babble*

■ Begins to search for a dropped toy within the visual field (emerging *permanence of object*)

Posture and large movements

■ Lying on back, raises head up and moves arms up to be lifted.

■ When hands grasped, braces shoulders and pulls self to sitting.

■ Sits with support with head and back straight and turns head from side to side to look around. (Independent sitting without support is achieved at 7 months (5–9 months.)

■ Can roll over from front to back (prone to supine) at around 5–6 months and usually from back to front (supine to prone) a little later at around 6–7 months.

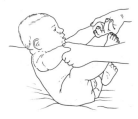

pulls self to sitting, braces shoulders

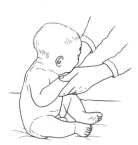

held sitting, back straight

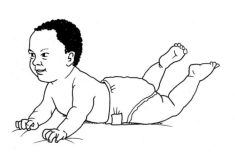

lying on abdomen, arms extended

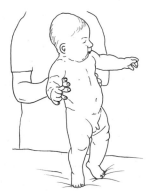

held standing, takes weight on legs

Table 1 Protective reflexes.

These reflexes develop from 4 to 5 months onwards and can be absent or abnormal in motor disorders.

Downward parachute reflex	5–6 months	When held and rapidly lowered the infant extends and abducts both legs and feet are plantigrade.
Sideward protective reflex	6–7 months	Infant puts arms out to save if tilted off balance.
Forward protective reflex	7–9 months	Arms and hands extend on forward descent to ground.
Backward protective reflex	8–9 months	Backward protective extension of both arms when pushed backwards in sitting position.

Source: Milani-Comparetti and Gidoni (1967).

- Placed on abdomen, lifts head and chest well up, supporting self on extended arms and flattened palms (4–8 months).

- Bears weight on feet and bounces up and down actively when held in supported standing with feet touching hard surface. Protective reflexes begin to appear (see Table 1).

Visual perceptual and fine motor development

- Visually insatiable: moves head and eyes eagerly in every direction when attention is distracted. Eyes move in unison. Follows adult's or child's activities across room with purposeful alertness. Immediately stares at interesting small objects or toys within 15–30 centimetres. Shows awareness of depth.

- Stretches out both hands simultaneously to grasp. Uses hands competently to reach for and grasp small toys. Mainly uses two-handed scooping-in approach, but will occasionally use a single hand. Adjusts arm and hand posture to orientation of the object. Uses whole hand to palmar grasp and passes toy from one hand to another. Drops one object if another is offered.

- When toy falls from hand within visual field, watches to resting place. When toy falls outside visual field, searches vaguely around with eyes and hands (early permanence of object), or forgets it.

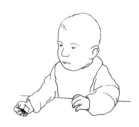

palmar grasp

Cognitive development: Understanding of the physical world – permanence of object

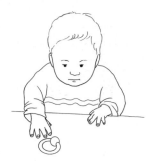

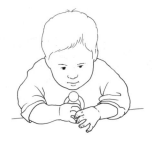

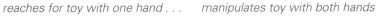

reaches for toy with one hand . . .   manipulates toy with both hands

Hearing behaviour

- Turns immediately to a familiar voice across the room.

- Listens to voice even if adult not in view.

- Turns to source when hears sounds at ear level.

Speech, language and communication

Stages of speech sound development

- Vocalises tunefully to self and others, using sing-song vowel sounds or single and double syllables, e.g. 'a-a', 'muh', 'goo', 'der', 'adah', 'er-leh', 'aroo' (4–8 months).

- Laughs, chuckles and squeals aloud in play. Screams with annoyance.

- Shows recognition of carer's facial expressions such as *happy* or *fearful* and responds selectively to emotional tones of voice.

Social behaviour and play

- Shows delighted response to rough-and-tumble play. Reacts enthusiastically to often-repeated games. Shows anticipation responses if carer pauses before high points in nursery rhymes and other action songs.

- Follows adult pointing towards an object or a person. Toys can be the shared focus of play.

- When offered a rattle, reaches for it immediately and shakes deliberately to make a sound, often regarding it closely at the same time. Manipulates objects attentively, passing them frequently from hand to hand. Takes everything to mouth. When totally absorbed in exploration of objects, may seem oblivious to carer's attempts to engage in interaction.

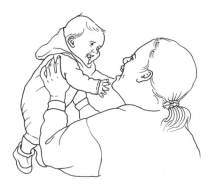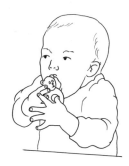

shows delighted response to rough-and-tumble play

takes everything to mouth

■ Still friendly with strangers but occasionally shows some shyness or even slight anxiety when approached too closely or abruptly, especially if familiar adult is out of sight. Becomes more reserved with strangers from around 7 months.

■ Places hand on breast while feeding, or if fed with formula milk, puts hand on bottle and pats it. May attempt to grasp cup if used.

■ Beginning to take smooth semi-solids. Initially spits out food using back-and-forth tongue movements. Gradually learns to suck food from spoon.

Self-care and independence

Isla

Non-verbal and social development

Isla

Gross motor: Neuro-motor examination

Isla

Social communication and play

AGE 9 MONTHS

Key developmental milestones

- Pulls to stand from sitting

- Index finger approach and pincer grasp of small objects

- Looks for fallen or hidden (in sight) objects – *permanence of object*

- Shows causal understanding (cause and effect) and means–end relations

- *Babbles* tunefully and communicatively

- Shows *stranger wariness*

- Plays social games, e.g. peek-a-boo and pat-a-cake

Posture and large movements

- Pulls self to sitting position. Sits unsupported on the floor and can adjust body posture when leaning forward to pick up and manipulate a toy without losing balance.

- Can turn body to look sideways while stretching out to pick up toy from floor.

- Progresses on floor by rolling, wriggling on abdomen or crawling from 7 months (5–11 months).

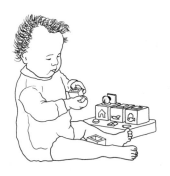

sits on floor and manipulates toys

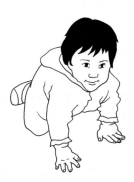

attempts to crawl

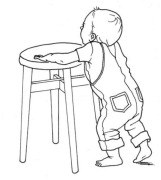

pulls to standing

- Pulls to standing (7–12 months), holding on to support for a few moments but cannot lower self and falls backwards with a bump.

- Held standing, steps purposefully on alternate feet.

- Only needs intermittent support when sitting on parent's or carer's lap and being dressed. When being carried by an adult, supports self in upright position and turns head to look around.

- Visually very attentive to people, objects and happenings in the environment.

Visual perceptual and fine motor

- Most fundamental visual functions, such as depth perception for working out the relative position of objects in visual field, and smooth visual attention to moving objects, are now in place.

- Immediately stretches out to grasp a small toy when offered, with one hand leading. Manipulates toy with a lively interest, passing from hand to hand and turning over.

- Regards unoffered but accessible toy before grasping, especially if unfamiliar.

- Can reach and grasp a moving object by moving towards the anticipated position of the moving object.

- Pokes at small object with index finger and begins to point at more distant object with same finger.

- Grasps string between finger and thumb in scissor fashion in order to pull toy towards self.

- Picks up small object between finger and thumb with 'inferior' pincer grasp.

- Can release toy from grasp by dropping or pressing against a firm surface but cannot yet release smoothly.

- Enjoys casting objects over the side of cot or chair.

- Looks in correct direction for falling or fallen toys (permanence of object).

Cognitive
development:
Understanding of
the physical world –
causal relationships

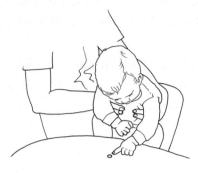

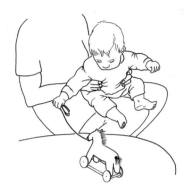

pokes at small objects using index finger   *grasps string to pull toy*

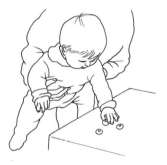

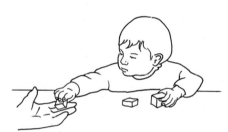

picks up small object with pincer grasp   *attempts to give block, but cannot yet release*

- Shows understanding of things that are causally connected, e.g. plays with cause-and-effect toys and pulls on a string to get the connected toy (early causal understanding).

- Watches activities of people or animals within 3 or 4 metres with sustained interest for several minutes.

Hearing behaviour

- Eagerly attentive to everyday sounds, particularly voice.

- Turns to search and localise faint sounds on either side.

- Locates sounds made above and below ear level.

- Vocalises deliberately as a means of interpersonal communication – in friendliness or annoyance. Shouts to attract attention, listens, then shouts again.

- Babbles loudly and tunefully in long repetitive strings of syllables, e.g. 'dad-dad', 'mum-mum', 'ababa', 'agaga'. *Babble* is practised largely for self-amusement, but also within 'conversations' with carers (7–9 months).

- Responds when name is called (6–10 months).

- Gaze-switching – looks between objects and people.

- Understands 'no!' and 'bye-bye' (6 –9 months).

- Reacts to 'where's mummy/daddy?' by looking around.

- Imitates playful vocal and other sounds, e.g. smacking lips, cough, 'brrr'.

Speech, language and communication

Speech sound development

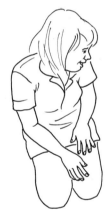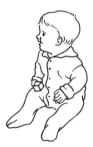

turns to sound, such as when name is called

Note: The vocalisations of children with severely impaired hearing remain at the primitive level and do not usually progress to repetitive tuneful babble. Poor or monotonous vocalisations after 8 or 9 months of age should always arouse suspicion.

Social behaviour and play

- Throws body back and stiffens in annoyance or resistance, usually protesting vocally at same time.

- Clearly distinguishes strangers from familiars and requires reassurance before accepting their advances; clings to known person and hides face (from 7 months).

- Still takes everything to mouth.

- Grasps bell by handle and rings in imitation. Shakes a rattle, explores it with a finger and bangs on floor.

- Plays 'peek-a-boo' and imitates hand-clapping.

- Offers food to familiar people and animals.

- Grasps toy in hand and offers to adult but cannot yet give into adult's hand.

- Offers/shows objects to enlist others in interaction.

- Watches toy being partially hidden under a cover or cup, and then finds it. May find toy wholly hidden under cushion or cup.

- Sustained interest for up to full minute in looking at pictures named by adult.

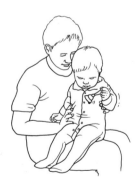

grasps bell by hands and rings in imitation

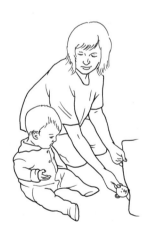

watches while toy is partly hidden . . .

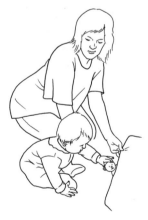

. . . and promptly finds toy

■ Holds, bites and chews small pieces of food.

■ Puts hands on breast or around bottle or cup when drinking.

■ Tries to grasp spoon when being fed.

■ Enjoys babbling with a mouthful of food.

Self-care and independence

AGE 12 MONTHS

Key developmental milestones

■ Independent walking emerges

■ Mature finger grasp

■ Initiating *joint attention*

■ Following simple instructions associated with gestures

Posture and large movements

■ Sits on floor for indefinite time. Can rise to sitting position from lying down with ease.

■ Crawls on hands and knees, shuffles on buttocks or 'bearwalks' rapidly about the floor. May crawl upstairs.

■ Pulls to standing and sits down again, holding onto furniture.

■ Walks around furniture lifting one foot and stepping sideways. May stand alone for a few moments (9–16 months).

■ Walks forwards and sideways with one or both hands held. May walk alone (9½–17½ months).

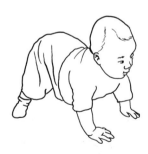

bearwalks around floor

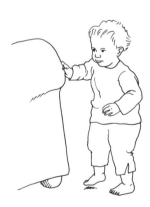

cruises, holding onto furniture

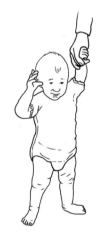

walks with one hand held

Visual perceptual and fine motor

■ When outside, watches movement of people, animals or motor vehicles for prolonged periods.

■ Recognises familiar people approaching from a distance.

■ Shows interest in pictures.

■ Has a mature grasp. Picks up small objects with neat pincer grasp between thumb and tip of index finger. By 13 months, reaching and grasping become coordinated into one smooth action, e.g. closing of hand starts during approach and well before touching the object.

■ Can release a cube/toy gently to give. Builds tower of two cubes after demonstration by 13 months (11–18 months).

■ Deliberately drops and throws toys forwards and watches them fall to the ground. Looks in correct place for toys that fall out of sight.

■ Points with index finger at objects of interest.

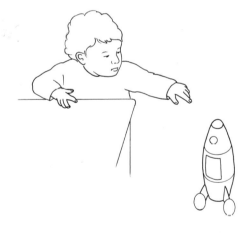

points with index finger to objects of interest

■ Begins to search in several locations for a hidden object (12–18 months).

■ Uses both hands freely but may show preference for one. Holds two toy bricks, one in each hand with tripod grasp, and bangs together to make noise.

Development of joint attention

Hearing behaviour

■ Locates sounds from any direction well. Responds immediately to own name.

■ Shows recognition of familiar songs by trying to join in.

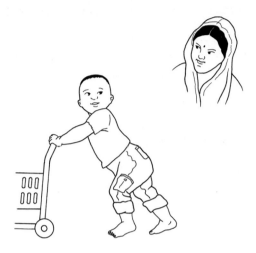

responds immediately to own name

Speech, language and communication

■ Babbles loudly and incessantly in conversational cadences (*jargon*). Vocalisation contains most vowels and many consonants.

■ Shows by behaviour that some words are understood in usual context, e.g. car, drink, cat. Understands simple instructions associated with a gesture, e.g. 'Give it to Daddy', 'Come to Mummy' (8–12 months).

■ Frequently responds to familiar songs by vocalising. Imitates adult playful vocalisations, e.g. 'uh-oh', and may use a few words, although with inconsistent pronunciation (12–15 months).

■ Will follow the gaze of an adult. Points to objects and then looks back to the adult for a reaction, in order to make a request or to elicit a comment from the adult.

COMPANION @ WEBSITE

Theories of language learning

Social behaviour and play

■ Takes objects to mouth less often. Very little, if any, drooling of saliva other than when eating, mouthing toys or when tired (12–18 months).

- Will put objects in and out of cup or box when shown.

- Likes to be in sight and hearing of familiar people. Demonstrates affection to familiars.

- Plays 'pat-a-cake' and waves 'good-bye', both on request and spontaneously.

- Enjoys joint play with adults, actively switching attention between objects and adult (coordinated *joint attention*).

- Manipulates toys and will shake to make noise. Listens with pleasure to sound-making toys and repeats appropriate activity (e.g. presses button) to reproduce sound.

- Gives toys to adults on request and sometimes spontaneously.

Development of joint attention

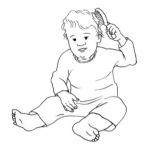

definition-by-use of everyday objects

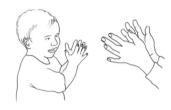

plays 'pat-a-cake'

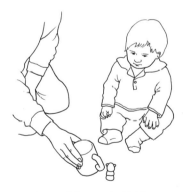

watches while toy is hidden under cup

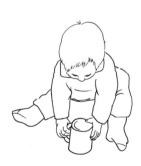

lifts cup to search for the toy

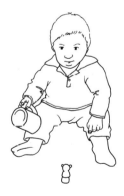

promptly finds toy, and looks to adult

■ Demonstrates understanding by use of objects, e.g. hairbrush, telephone (*definition-by-use*).

■ Quickly finds toys hidden from view.

Self-care and independence

■ Drinks well from a lidded cup with little assistance.

■ Holds spoon and will attempt to use for feeding, although very messy.

■ Munches pieces of food at sides of mouth.

■ Sits, or sometimes stands, without support while dressed by carer.

■ Helps with dressing by holding out arm for sleeve and foot for shoe.

From Birth to Five Years – Practical Developmental Examination

Clinical evaluation

Ruby

Non-verbal and social development

Ruby

Social communication and play

BOX 1 Variability in motor milestones

Development does not progress at the same rate in all children – there is broad variation in 'typical' ages of achieving milestones. Most children, however, follow a similar pattern or sequence of development. In some situations, depending on the child, family or environment-related factors, an 'atypical' sequence or pattern may be present along with different rate of progress. Children's progress to walking independently is one such example:

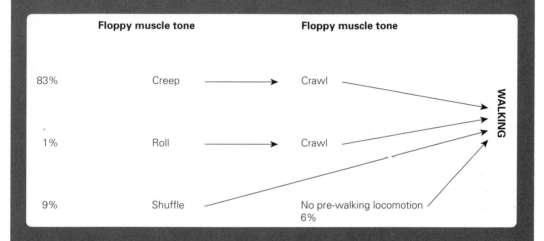

Eighty percent of children sit independently between 7 months (mean age) and 11 months (97th centile) and walk between 13 months (mean age) and 18 months (97th centile). Around 9 per cent of children don't crawl before walking but do shuffle on their bottom, often with a family history of bottom shuffling and/or low muscle tone. These children are also very late in independent sitting (12 months mean age, 15 months 97th centile) and independent walking (17 months mean age and 24 months 97th centile). There is small group of children (1 per cent) who skip crawling or shuffling altogether and go straight to independent walking, slightly before the rest of their peer group (11 months mean age and 14 months 97th centile). All three groups have normal patterns. However, a neurological examination is recommended for those who are not walking by 18 months of age to exclude any disorder.

AGE 15 MONTHS

Key developmental milestones

- Independent walking
- Mature release of objects – makes tower of two cubes
- First words
- Functional use of toys

Posture and large movements

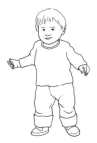

walks independently, feet apart, arms assisting balance

- May walk alone, usually with uneven steps: feet wide apart, arms slightly flexed and held above head or at shoulder level for balance (9½–17½ months). Walks with broad base, high-stepping *gait* and steps of unequal length. Starts voluntarily but frequently stopped by falling or bumping into furniture.

- Note: infants who 'bottom shuffle' are usually delayed in walking (17–28 months).

- Lets self down from standing to sitting by collapsing backward with a bump, or by falling forwards on hands and then back to sitting. Can get back to feet alone.

- Creeps upstairs safely and may get downstairs backwards.

- Kneels unaided or with support.

Visual perceptual and fine motor

- Watches small toy pulled across floor. Demands desired objects out of reach by pointing with index finger. Stands at window and watches outside happenings with interest. Attends to coloured pictures in book and pats page.

- Picks up string or small objects with a precise pincer grasp, using either hand.

- Manipulates cubes and may build a tower of two cubes after demonstration from 13 months (11–18 months). Can take objects out of container and replace fairly precisely, e.g. pegs in holes.

- Grasps crayon with whole hand, using palmar grasp. Uses either hand and imitates to-and-fro scribble from 14 months (11–18 months).

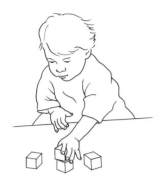

manipulates blocks and builds tower of two

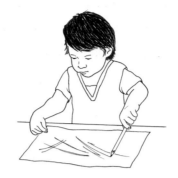

grasps crayon with whole hand and scribbles to and fro

■ Uses *jargon*, with intonation patterns that sound like connected speech.

■ Says a few recognisable words (usually a range of between two and six) spontaneously in correct context (12–18 months).

■ Appears to understand some new words each week.

■ Will sustain interest for two or more minutes in looking at pictures during shared book reading.

■ Understands and obeys simple, familiar instructions, such as 'Don't touch', 'Come for dinner', 'Give me the ball'.

■ Points to familiar persons, animals or toys when requested.

■ Communicates wishes and needs by pointing and vocalising or screaming.

Speech, language and communication

■ Pushes large, wheeled toy with handle on level ground.

■ Explores properties and possibilities of toys, convenient household objects and sound-makers with lively interest.

■ Engages in functional play, e.g. pushing toy car, pretends to drink from empty cup, bangs with toy hammer, etc.

■ Carries dolls by limbs, hair or clothing. Repeatedly casts objects to floor, in play or rejection, and watches where things fall. Looks for hidden toy.

Social behaviour and play

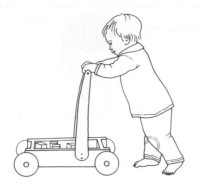 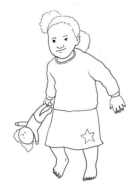

pushes large wheeled toy on level ground   *likes carrying toy/doll*

■ Enjoys 'give and take' games, including initiating teasing by offering and then withdrawing an object. Physically restless and intensely curious regarding people, objects and events.

■ Points to share interest – *joint attention* (12–18 months).

■ Emotionally labile and closely dependent upon adult's reassuring presence. Looks to caregiver to monitor his/her reactions, particularly in unfamiliar situations (*social referencing*). Is affectionate to familiar people.

Self-care and independence

■ Holds and drinks from a cup.

■ Attempts to hold spoon, brings it to mouth and licks it but is unlikely to prevent it turning over.

■ Competent finger feeding. Chews well but continues to spill from mouth as lip closure is not maintained.

■ Helps more constructively with dressing.

■ Needs constant supervision for protection against dangers owing to extended exploration of the environment.

AGE 18 MONTHS

Key developmental milestones

- Emerging hand preference

- Says a range of single words

- Follows simple situational directions, shows body parts

- Awareness of self-identity

- Early symbolic play: use of toys or doll/others

- Acts out familiar actions in play

- Imitating day-to-day activities at home

- Walks well with feet only slightly apart, starts and stops safely.

- No longer needs to hold upper arms in extension to balance.

- Runs rather carefully and stiffly, though seldom falls; head held erect in midline, eyes fixed on ground 1–2 metres ahead but finds difficulty in negotiating obstacles.

- Pushes and pulls large toys or boxes along the floor.

- Can carry large doll or teddy bear while walking. Backs into small chair or slides in sideways to seat self.

- Enjoys climbing and will climb forwards into adult's chair, then turn round and sit.

- Walks upstairs with helping hand from 16 months (13–22 months) and sometimes downstairs.

- Creeps backwards downstairs or occasionally bumps down a few steps on buttocks facing forwards.

- Kneels upright on flat surface without support. Flexes knees and hips in squatting position to pick up toy from floor and rises to feet using hands as support (15–18 months).

Posture and large movements

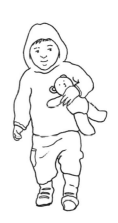

walks well carrying toy

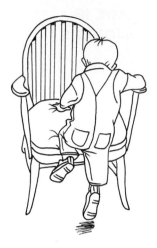

climbs into adult chair

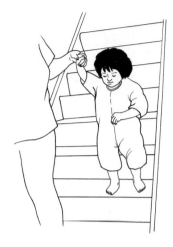

walks up and down stairs with help

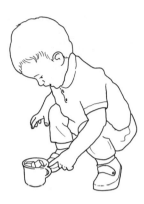

squats to pick up toy

Visual perceptual and fine motor

■ Picks up small objects immediately on sight with delicate pincer grasp. Recognises familiar people at a distance and points to distant interesting objects when outdoors.

■ Enjoys simple picture books, often recognising and putting index finger on boldly coloured items on page. Turns several pages at a time.

■ Holds pencil in mid- or upper shaft in whole hand in a pronated grip, or with crude approximation of thumb and fingers. Spontaneous to-and-fro scribble and dots, using either hand alone or sometimes with pencils in both hands.

■ Builds tower of three cubes after demonstration and sometimes spontaneously. Enjoys placing small objects in and out of containers and learning the relative size of objects.

■ Emerging understanding of other person's intentions and desires from their expressions and actions (18–24 months).

■ Beginning to show preference for using either the right or the left hand.

Development of social understanding

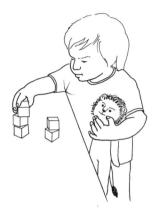

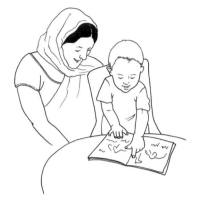

builds tower of three blocks   *enjoys picture books*

■ Chatters continually to self during play, with conversational intonation and emotional inflections (mix of *jargon* and intelligible
words).

■ Listens and responds to spoken communications addressed
directly to self. Uses between six and twenty recognisable
words and understands many more. Echoes prominent or last
word in short sentences addressed to self. Growth spurt in
spoken vocabulary from 18 months (18–24 months]).

■ Demands a desired object by pointing accompanied by loud,
urgent vocalisations or single words, checking back to adult that
request has been noted.

■ Enjoys nursery rhymes and tries to join in. Attempts to sing.

■ Hands familiar objects to adult when requested (even if more
than one option available). Obeys simple instructions, e.g. 'get
your shoes' or 'shut the door'. Points to own, carer's or doll's
hair, shoes, nose, feet.

■ Explores environment energetically and with increasing understanding. Poor self-control and low risk-awareness requires
constant supervision.

■ No longer takes toys to mouth.

**Speech,
language and
communication**

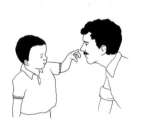

*points to person's
nose*

**Social behaviour
and play**

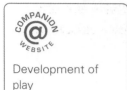

Development of play

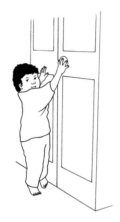

explores environment

■ Remembers where objects belong in familiar environments.

■ Still casts objects to floor in play or anger, but less often, and seldom troubles to check where object has landed.

■ Fascinated by household objects and imitates simple, everyday activities such as feeding doll, reading book, brushing floor, washing clothes ('domestic mimicry' or 'deferred imitation') (15–18 months).

■ Acts out familiar routines in play, e.g. handing out cups in tea party. Treats dolls and teddies as babies, e.g. hugging, feeding, putting to bed, etc.

■ Rigid attention to tasks of own choosing. Resistance to interference.

■ Plays contentedly alone but likes to be near familiar adult or older sibling. Emotionally still very dependent upon familiar adult, alternating between clinging and resistance.

■ Recognises self in a mirror.

■ Exchanges toys, both cooperatively and in conflict, with peers.

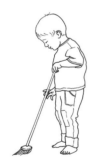

imitates everyday activities

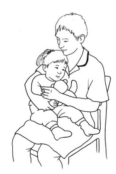

still dependent upon familiar adult

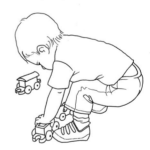

plays contentedly alone

■ Holds spoon and gets food safely to mouth, although may play with food. Holds cup between both hands and drinks without much spilling. Lifts cup alone but usually hands back to adult when finished.

■ Assists with dressing and undressing, taking off shoes, socks and hat, but seldom able to replace.

■ Beginning to give notice of urgent toilet needs by restlessness and vocalisation. Bowel control may be attained but very variable. May indicate wet or soiled pants.

Self-care and independence

AGE 2 YEARS

> **Key developmental milestones**
>
> ■ Runs safely
>
> ■ Typically uses two-word combinations
>
> ■ Follows two-step instructions
>
> ■ Does circular scribble with a crayon/pencil
>
> ■ Mostly uses preferred hand
>
> ■ Turns pages of a book singly

Posture and large movements

■ Runs safely on whole foot, stopping and starting with ease and avoiding obstacles.

■ Squats with complete steadiness to rest or to play with an object on the ground and rises to feet without using hands.

■ Jumps in place after demonstration (17–30 months).

■ Pushes and pulls large, wheeled toys easily forwards and usually able to walk backwards pulling handle. Pulls small wheeled toy by cord with obvious appreciation of direction.

■ Climbs on furniture to look out of window or to open doors and can get down again.

■ Shows increasing understanding of size of self in relation to size and position of objects in the environment and to enclosed spaces such as a cupboard or cardboard box.

■ Walks upstairs and downstairs holding on to rail or wall, two feet to a step.

■ Throws small ball overhand and forwards, without falling over.

■ Walks into large ball when trying to kick it.

■ Sits on small tricycle but cannot use pedals. Propels vehicle forwards with feet on floor.

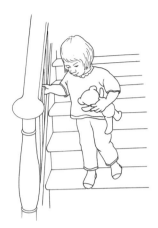

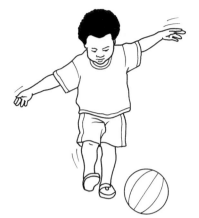

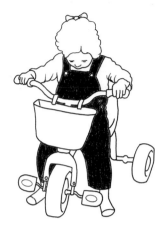

walks up and down stairs

walks into large ball

sits and steers tricycle, cannot yet use pedals

- Good manipulative skills; picks up tiny objects accurately and quickly and places down neatly with increasing skill.

- Can match square, circular and triangular shapes in a simple jigsaw.

- Holds a pencil well down shaft towards point, using thumb and first two fingers. Mostly uses preferred hand.

- Spontaneous circular scribble as well as to-and-fro scribble and dots; imitates vertical line and sometimes 'V' shape.

- Builds tower of six or seven cubes.

- Enjoys picture books, recognising fine details in favourite pictures. Turns pages singly. Can name and match pictures with toys or with other pictures.

- Recognises self and familiar adults in photographs.

- Binocular vision at this age can be tested with Kay Pictures Vision Test.

Visual perceptual and fine motor

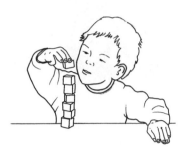

builds tower of six or seven blocks

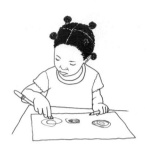

holds pencil and scribbles

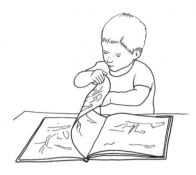

enjoys books, turns pages singly

Speech, language and communication

■ Uses fifty or more recognisable words appropriately and understands many more. Puts two or more words together to form simple sentences (18–30 months). Starting to use 'no' and 'not'. Constantly asking names of objects and people. May omit sounds or parts of words.

■ Attends to communications addressed to self, although may need prompt to stop and shift attention. Begins to listen with obvious interest to more general conversation.

■ Refers to self by name or using personal pronoun (me) and talks to self continually in long monologues during play but may be incomprehensible to others.

■ *Echolalia* almost constant, with one or more stressed words repeated.

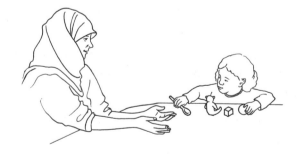

hands familiar objects to adults on request

■ Joins in nursery rhymes and action songs.

■ Indicates hair, hand, feet, nose, eyes, mouth, shoes, etc. in pictures. Names familiar objects and pictures.

■ Carries out simple instructions such as 'Go and see what the postman has brought'. Follows a series of two simple but related commands, e.g. 'Get your teddy and put it in the bag'.

■ Can select a named object from a display of three or four objects.

■ Follows parent or carer around house and imitates domestic activities in simultaneous play. Intensely curious regarding environment. Turns door handles and often runs outside. Little comprehension of common dangers.

Social behaviour and play

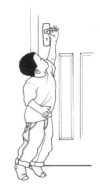

■ Spontaneously engages in simple role or situational make-believe activities. Beginning to show meaningful short play sequences, and *definition-by-use* of doll's-house-sized toys. Substitutes one item for another, e.g. pretends a brick is a car or a banana is a telephone (18–24 months).

■ Understands that others may have desires that differ from their own.

■ Constantly demanding parent's or carer's attention. Clings tightly in affection, fatigue or fear, although resistive and rebellious when thwarted. Tantrums when frustrated or when trying to make self understood, but attention is usually readily distracted.

turns door handle, has little comprehension of dangers

■ Defends own possessions with determination.

■ May take turns but, as yet, has little idea of sharing either toys or the attention of adults.

■ Parallel play present; plays contentedly near other children but not with them. Beginning to cooperate with sibling/peer to achieve a goal.

■ Resentful of attention shown to other children, particularly by own familiars.

■ Unwilling to defer or modify immediate satisfaction of wishes.

COMPANION @ WEBSITE

Development of play

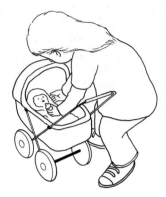

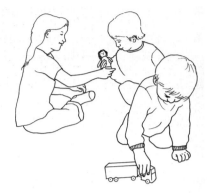

engages in make-believe play *plays near others but not with them*

Self-care and independence

■ Feeds self competently with a spoon but is easily distracted. Controlled biting on biscuits. Chews with lips closed, some spillage.

■ Lifts open cup and drinks well without spilling and replaces cup on table without difficulty. Asks for food and drink.

■ Usually attempts to verbalise toilet needs in reasonable time, but still unreliable.

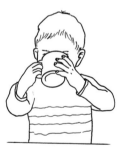

lifts cup and drinks well without spillage

BOX 2 Variation in language milestones

The variation in language acquisition between individuals, in relation to both rate and learning style, is pertinent to the questions of how to identify children who are delayed, and which children may go on to have disorders. The range of variation in ages at which children achieve language milestones is greater than variation in other domains of development as language development is subject to the complex interplay between a wide range of genetic and environmental factors. Areas studied have included the age at which children acquire word comprehension, production of first words, and the transition to word combinations.

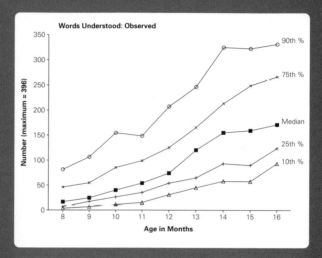

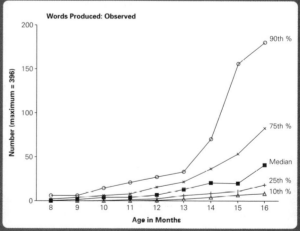

The figures right (Fenson *et al*. 1994) illustrate the range in the number of words understood and the number of words produced, in a sample of children aged between 8 and 16 months, on a parental report questionnaire (Fenson *et al*. 1993). Similar results have been found in laboratory studies. In the figures right, at the age of 11 months, the 'average range' (i.e. 80 per cent of children)

includes '10 words understood' to '144 words understood'. Expressive vocabulary development may show a dramatic increase from 12 months onwards, but the 'average range' includes children with fewer than ten words at 16 months. Such children are often referred to as 'late talkers', who, in the absence of other risk factors, usually catch up with the rest of their peer group within a year.

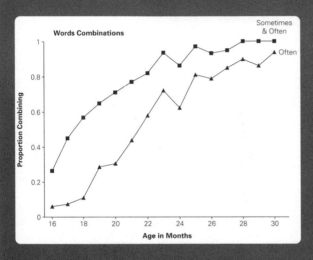

The figure left (Fenson *et al.* 1994) represents the percentage of children producing short phrases. Consistent correlations between expressive vocabulary size and the emergence of word combinations (typically between 50 and 100 words) have been found. Variability in vocabulary growth contributes to variation in word combinations, with a steep rise in the number of children using word combinations until around 24 months of age. The majority of children have achieved this milestone by 30 months.

As a rule of thumb, infants who are not demonstrating any word recognition at 12 months, not using any recognisable words at 18 months, not demonstrating vocabulary growth beyond 50 words by 2 years, or not combining words at 2½ years may be a cause for concern. The decision as to whether to instigate further assessment, or offer support, will be dependent on the presence of genetic, medical or environmental risk factors, the child's developmental profile in other domains (motor, cognitive, etc.) and the degree of parental concern.

Louisa

Non-verbal and
social development

Louisa

Social
communication
and play

Louisa

Gross motor
skills

*From Birth to Five
Years – Practical
Developmental
Examination*

Clinical evaluation

AGE 2½ YEARS

Key developmental milestones

■ Jumps with two feet together

■ Throws and kicks a ball

■ Draws a circle in imitation

■ Uses pronouns 'I' and 'you'

■ Understands action words

■ Provides a verbal commentary during play

Posture and large movements

■ Runs well and climbs easy nursery apparatus. Walks upstairs confidently and downstairs holding rail, two feet to a step.

■ Pushes and pulls large toys skilfully but may have difficulty in steering them around obstacles.

■ Can jump with two feet together from a low step. Can stand and walk on tiptoe if shown (16–30 months).

■ Throws ball from hand somewhat stiffly at body level. Kicks large ball but gently and lopsidedly.

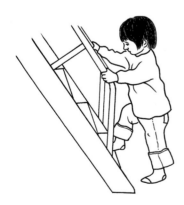

climbs play equipment

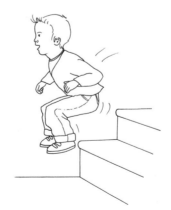

jumps from bottom step, both feet together

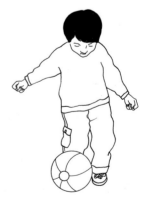

kicks large ball gently

■ Recognises minute details in picture books. Recognises self in photographs once shown.

■ Begins to respond to social information on TV and other media as relevant to everyday experiences.

■ Builds tower of seven-plus cubes using preferred hand. Inserts square, circular and triangular shapes in a jigsaw by recognising the shape. Begins to correct the orientation of the shapes from 33 months.

■ Holds pencil in preferred hand, with improved tripod grasp.

■ Imitates horizontal line and circle, and usually 'T' and 'V'.

■ Matches 3–4 colours correctly (24–36 months).

■ Uses 200 or more recognisable words (24–36 months), but speech shows numerous immaturities of articulation and sentence structure.

■ Usually intelligible to familiar carers.

■ Knows full name.

■ Talks audibly and intelligibly to self at play, concerning events happening here and now.

■ Continues to imitate phrases (echolalia).

■ Can select pictures of actions, e.g. 'Which one is eating?' (24–33 months).

■ Recognises general family name categories, e.g. 'baby', 'mother', 'granny', etc.

■ Makes frequent comments on objects and events of interest, directed to caregivers.

■ Continually asking questions beginning 'What?' or 'Who?'. Uses pronouns 'I', 'me' and 'you' correctly.

■ Stuttering in eagerness common.

■ Recites a few nursery rhymes.

Visual perceptual and fine motor

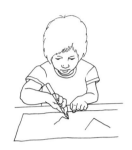

holds pencil in preferred hand and imitates 'v'

Speech, language and communication

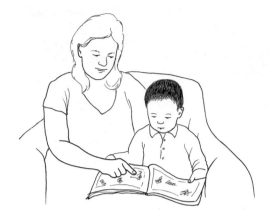

enjoys simple familiar stories in picture books

■ Enjoys simple familiar stories read from picture book.

■ Provides a running commentary during play – to self or others.

■ Requires physical or verbal prompts in order to switch attention to looking and listening if engrossed in play.

Social behaviour and play

■ Exceedingly active, restless and resistive of restraint. Has little understanding of common dangers or need to defer immediate wishes.

■ Throws tantrums when thwarted and is less easily distracted.

■ Emotionally still very dependent on adult and requires reassurance in unfamiliar situations.

■ More sustained role play, such as putting dolls to bed, washing clothes, driving cars, but with frequent reference to a friendly adult.

■ Plays meaningfully with miniature doll's-house-sized toys.

■ Acts out common activities using substituted materials, e.g. has pretend tea parties, with gravel on plates to represent food.

■ Watches other children at play with interest, occasionally joining in for a few minutes but, as yet, has little notion of the necessity to share playthings or adults' attention.

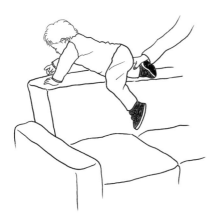

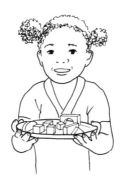

active and curious with little notion of common dangers

imaginative play, using substituted materials

Self-care and independence

■ Eats skilfully with spoon and may use a fork.

■ Pulls down pants when using the toilet but seldom is able to replace them.

■ May be dry through the night, although this is extremely variable.

AGE 3 YEARS

Key developmental milestones

■ Walks up stairs with alternating feet

■ Cuts with toy scissors

■ Holds a pencil near the point and copies circle

■ Asks 'what?', 'where?', 'who?' and 'why?' questions

■ Matches colours

■ Joins in *make-believe play* with other children

Posture and large movements

■ Walks alone up stairs using alternating feet, one foot to each step, comes down stairs two feet to a step and can carry large toy. Usually jumps from bottom step with two feet together.

■ Climbs nursery apparatus with agility.

■ Can turn around obstacles and corners while running and also while pushing and pulling large toys.

■ Walks forwards, backwards, sideways, etc., hauling large toys with confidence.

■ Obviously appreciates size and movements of own body in relation to external objects and space.

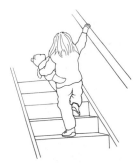

walks up and down stairs, carrying large toy

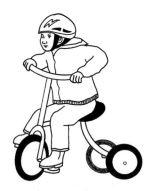

rides tricycle, using pedals

■ Rides tricycle using pedals and can steer it round wide corners.

■ Can stand and walk on tiptoe. Can stand momentarily on one (preferred) foot when shown.

■ Can sit with feet crossed at ankles.

■ Can throw a ball overhand and catch large ball on or between extended arms. Kicks ball forcibly.

■ Builds tower of nine or ten cubes; builds a four-brick train with a chimney (33–42 months) and by 3½ years builds one or more bridges of three cubes from a model using two hands cooperatively. Threads large wooden beads on shoelace (not by pattern).

Visual perceptual and fine motor

■ Holds pencil near the point in preferred hand, between the first two fingers and thumb, and uses it with good control. Copies circle, also letters 'V', 'H' and 'T'. Imitates a cross. Draws person with head and usually adds one or two other features or parts.

Development of drawing skills

■ Can close fist and wiggle thumb in imitation, right and left.

■ Matches two or three primary colours, usually red and yellow, but may confuse blue and green. May know names of colours.

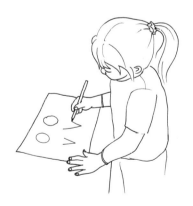

copies circle and letter 'v'

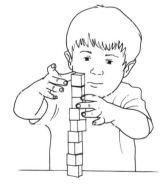

builds tower of nine or ten blocks

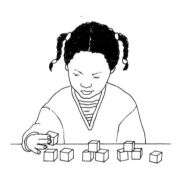

builds three-block bridges from a model

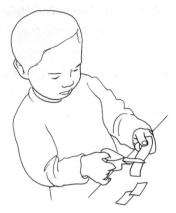

cuts with scissors

■ Enjoys painting with large brush on easel, covering whole paper with wash of colour or painting primitive 'pictures', which are usually named during or after production.

■ Understands visual perspective taking – would turn a picture around to show.

■ Cuts paper with toy scissors (neatly from 3½ to 4 years).

Speech, language and communication

■ Speech modulated in loudness and range of pitch. Large vocabulary intelligible even to strangers, but speech still contains many immature sound substitutions and simplified grammatical forms.

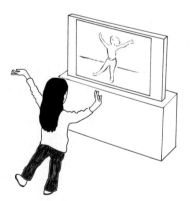

enjoys watching television, will join in action songs

- Gives full name and sex and, sometimes, age. Uses personal pronouns and plurals correctly, and also most prepositions.

- Still talks to self in long monologues, mostly concerned with the immediate present, particularly during make-believe activities. Carries on simple conversations and is able to describe briefly present activities and past experiences.

- Asks many questions beginning 'What?', 'Where? and 'Who?'.

- Can identify objects by function, e.g. 'Which one do we eat with?'. Understands descriptive concepts such as 'big', 'wet', 'hot', 'the same', etc.

- Listens eagerly to stories and demands favourites over and over again. Knows several nursery rhymes to repeat and sometimes sing.

- Counts by rote up to ten or more, but little appreciation of quantity beyond two or three.

- Some ability to switch between doing and listening. Needs to look at the speaker in order to listen.

Social behaviour and play

- General behaviour is more amenable – can be affectionate and confiding. Makes reference to emotions and can show empathy.

- Vividly realised *make-believe play*, including invented people and objects, in addition to familiar activities and events.

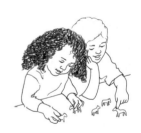

- Enjoys playing on the floor with bricks, boxes, toy trains and dolls, etc., alone or in company with siblings.

joins in make-believe play with other children

- Joins in active make-believe play with other children. Understands sharing playthings, but tends to pursue own ideas.

- Shows affection for younger siblings.

- Shows some appreciation of difference between present and past, and of the need to defer satisfaction of wishes to the future.

Self-care and independence

- Eats with a fork and spoon.

- Washes hands but needs adult supervision with drying. Can pull pants down and up but needs help with buttons and other fastenings.

- May be dry through the night, although this is very variable.

- Likes to help adults with domestic activities including gardening, shopping, etc.

- Makes an effort to keep surroundings tidy.

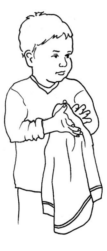

washes hands but needs supervision with drying

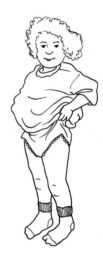

can pull pants down and up

Joshua

Non-verbal and social development

Joshua

Social communication and play

Joshua

Gross motor skills

AGE 4 YEARS

Key developmental milestones

■ Stands on one foot and hops

■ Holds a pencil in a dynamic tripod grasp, copies a cross and draws a person with head, trunk, legs, arms and, usually, fingers

■ Is able to relate recent experiences, using grammatical and intelligible sentences

■ Rote counts to twenty, counts objects to five

■ Shows sympathy for other children in distress

■ Recognises own name in print

■ Walks or runs alone up and down stairs, one foot to a step in adult fashion. Navigates self-locomotion skilfully, turning sharp corners, running, pushing and pulling.

Posture and large movements

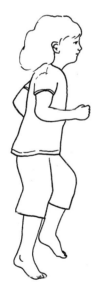 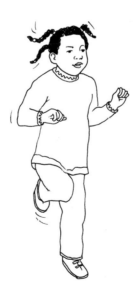 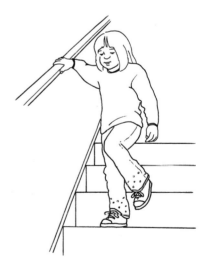

can stand or run on tiptoe   *hops on one foot*   *walks up and down stairs, one foot to a step*

■ Climbs ladders and trees.

■ Can stand, walk and run on tiptoe.

■ Expert rider of tricycle, executing sharp U-turns easily.

■ Stands on one (preferred) foot for 3–5 seconds and hops on preferred foot.

■ Arranges and picks up objects from floor by bending from waist with knees extended.

■ Sits with legs crossed.

■ Shows increasing skill in ball games, throwing, catching, bouncing, kicking, etc., including use of bat.

Visual perceptual and fine motor

■ Builds tower of ten or more cubes and several bridges of three from one model on request or spontaneously. Builds three steps with six cubes after demonstration (4–4½ years).

■ Imitates spreading of hand and bringing thumb into opposition with each finger in turn, right and left.

■ Holds and uses pencil in a dynamic tripod grasp with good control, like adults. Copies cross and also letters 'V', 'H', 'T' and 'O'.

■ Draws a person with head, legs and trunk and, usually, arms and fingers. Draws a recognisable house on request or spontaneously.

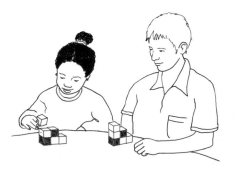
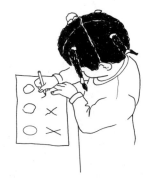

builds three steps after demonstration   *copies circles and crosses*

- Beginning to name drawings before production, and attempts to build with a range of materials, reflecting an ability to plan and execute ideas.

- Matches and names four primary colours correctly.

- Speech grammatically correct and completely intelligible. Shows only a few immature sound substitutions, usually of r-l-w-y group, p-th-f-s group or k-t sound group. May simplify consonant clusters, e.g. 'sring' for 'string'. Gives connected account of recent events and experiences. Gives full name, home address and usually age.

Speech, language and communication

- Continually asking questions 'Why?', 'When?', 'How?', and the meanings of words.

- Understands some abstract concepts, e.g. 'one of', 'before' and 'after', 'if'.

- Listens to and tells long stories, sometimes confusing fact and fantasy.

Cognitive development: Social understanding – Theory of Mind

- Counts by rote up to twenty or more, and beginning to count objects by word and touch in one-to-one correspondence up to four or five.

- Enjoys jokes and verbal incongruities.

- Knows several nursery rhymes and can repeat or sing correctly.

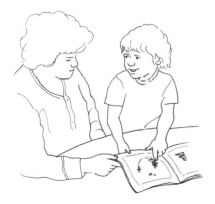

enjoys listening to and telling stories

Social behaviour and play

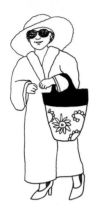

imaginative dressing-up play

■ General behaviour more independent and strongly self-willed. Adopts the standards of behaviour of parents or other close adults.

■ Inclined to verbal impertinence with adults and quarrelling with playmates when wishes crossed. May experiment with swearing/'rude words'.

■ Shows sense of humour in talk and social activities.

■ Dramatic *make-believe play* and dressing-up favoured. Floor games very complicated but habits less tidy.

■ Constructive outdoor building with any materials available.

■ Needs companionship of other children with whom he/she is alternately cooperative and aggressive, as with adults, but understands need to argue with words rather than blows. Understands taking turns as well as sharing.

■ Shows concern for younger siblings and sympathy for playmates in distress.

■ Appreciates past, present and future time.

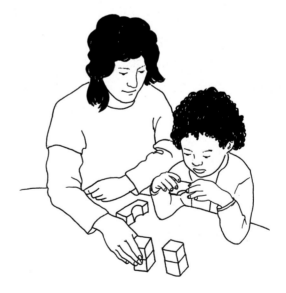

understands need for taking turns in play

- Eats skilfully with spoon and fork. Spreads butter on bread with a knife.

- Washes and dries hands. Brushes teeth. Can undress and dress except for laces, ties and back buttons (4–5 years).

Self-care and independence

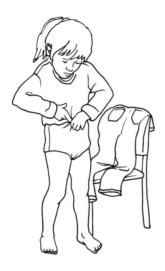

dresses and undresses alone

> **From Birth to Five Years – Practical Developmental Examination**
>
> Clinical evaluation

Alfie

Non-verbal and social development

Alfie

Social communication and play

Alfie

Gross motor skills

AGE 5 YEARS

Key developmental milestones

- Skilled in complex motor tasks, e.g. skipping, walking along a line

- Pencil skills for drawing a person, copying a triangle and colouring within outlines

- Can give name and age

- Able to engage in a to-and-fro conversation about a recent or routine past event

- Has a friend

Posture and large movements

- Walks easily on narrow line. Runs lightly on toes. Active and skilful in climbing, sliding, swinging, digging and doing various 'stunts'. Skips on alternate feet.

- Can stand on one foot for 8–10 seconds, right or left, and usually also stands on preferred foot, with arms folded. Can hop 2 or 3 metres forwards on each foot separately.

- Moves rhythmically to music.

- Grips strongly with either hand.

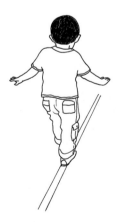

walks on narrow line

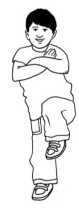

stands on one foot, arms folded

■ Can bend and touch toes without flexing knees.

■ Throws and catches a ball well, though catching with one hand does not develop until 9–10 years. Plays all varieties of ball games with considerable ability, including those requiring appropriate placement or scoring, according to accepted rules.

■ Picks up and replaces minute objects.

Visual perceptual and fine motor

■ Holds the cubes with the ulnar fingers tucked in and the hand diagonal to get a better view. Builds elaborate models when shown, such as three steps with six cubes from model; sometimes four steps from ten cubes (5–5½ years).

■ Good control in writing and drawing with pencils and paintbrushes. Copies square and, at 5½ years, a triangle. Also copies many letters such as 'V', 'T', 'H', 'O', 'X', 'L', 'A', 'C', 'U' and 'Y' with varying degree of accuracy. Writes a few letters spontaneously.

■ Draws recognisable man with head, trunk, legs, arms and features. Draws house with door, windows, roof and chimney.

■ Can cut a strip of paper neatly.

■ Spontaneously produces many other pictures containing several items and usually indication of background of environment, and names before production.

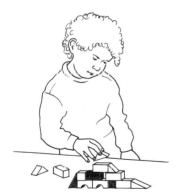
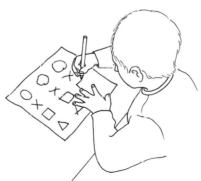

constructs elaborate models   *copies squares and triangles*

- Colours pictures neatly, staying within outlines.

- Counts fingers on one hand with index finger of other.

- Names four or more primary colours and matches ten or twelve colours.

Speech, language and communication

- Speech fluent, grammatically conventional and usually phonetically correct except for confusions of s-f-th group.

- Loves to be read or told stories and acts them out in detail later, alone or with friends.

- Gives full name, age and usually birthday. Gives home address.

- Can listen to instructions whilst engaged in activities.

- Defines concrete nouns by use.

- Understands time and sequence concepts and uses terms such as 'first', 'then', 'last'.

- Constantly asks meaning of abstract words and uses them, usually appropriately but with some errors.

- Delights in reciting or singing rhymes and jingles. Enjoys jokes and riddles.

Social behaviour and play

- Developing self-regulation. General behaviour more sensible, controlled and independent with wide variability in different situations. Able to hide/modulate emotions, and express socially appropriate responses to events.

- Follows tidiness routines but needs constant reminders.

- Domestic and dramatic play continued alone or with playmates from day to day. Enjoys stories about strong and powerful characters.

- Plays imaginatively, creating scenes using miniatures. Substitutes unrelated objects in play, e.g. pretends a brick is an apple.

- Plans and builds constructively in and outside.

- Chooses own friends. Can play cooperatively with peers most of the time and understands need for rules and fair play.

■ Increasing understanding of the feelings and wishes of friends, engaging in bargaining, compromise and reconciliation.

■ Shows definite sense of humour.

■ Appreciates meaning of time in relation to daily programme.

■ Tender and protective towards younger children and pets. Comforts playmates in distress.

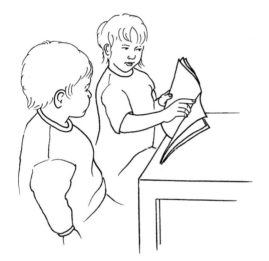

affectionate and helpful to younger children

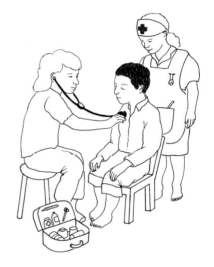

dramatic play with peers

■ Uses knife and fork competently.

■ Washes and dries face and hands but needs help or supervision for the rest. Undresses and dresses alone.

Self-care and independence

Domains of developmental progress

Section 2

Children's developmental progress

Child development is a *dynamic* process of growth, transformation, learning and acquisition of abilities to respond and adapt to the environment in a planned, organised and independent manner. This process does not simply unfold with neurological maturation but is shaped, positively or negatively, by the interactions between biological and environmental influences (Figure 1). These interactions result in a high level of variability in children's developmental outcomes. Learning about both the sequences of development and the context of development is necessary for understanding developmental progress.

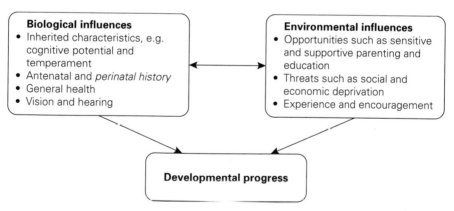

Figure 1 *Influences on development.*

Conventionally the study of child development is divided into domains, a convention that is followed within this volume. However, the divisions are somewhat artificial and driven by pragmatic considerations. There is only a broad agreement on the

Domains and sequences of development

names and definitions of domains, with a range of terms being used, e.g. posture and large movements (motor), visual perceptual and fine motor (eye and hand coordination, non-verbal performance, cognitive), language (speech, language and communication), self-help and independence (personal-social), social behaviour and play. While the core aspect of each domain has a distinct neuro-psychological basis, the domains overlap and are heavily inter-twined in their development and functional expression. All domains progress in an interconnected manner as part of a *dynamic* system. For example, children's fine motor function develops as part of a system which includes elements of posture and motor development, sensory modalities and cognitive abilities. Similarly, social behaviour is an integrated product of sensory, cognitive, linguistic and, at least to some degree, postural and fine motor abilities.

The overarching sequence in children's developmental progress consists of multiple cycles of progressive differentiation, integration and specialisation at neurological, psychological and behavioural levels. This is a self-organising and systematic process driven and refined by the interaction between *genetic expression*, neuro-psychological growth and environmental experience. As the child's sensory and exploratory abilities become refined and integrated, new experiences – physical and social – are created. The continually adaptive developmental processes lead to further refined levels of perception and responses, which in turn spur new genetic expressions. These ongoing interactions and cycles of progressive integration and reorganisation generate higher, and some qualitatively new, levels of physical, emotional, social, linguistic and cognitive ability.

Developmental milestones, stages and variations

Children's developmental milestones are convenient guidelines for looking at the rate or the extent of their progress. Even though the sequences of developmental milestones are similar in most children, there is a wide individual variation in the rate of achievement, largely attributable to the factors outlined in Figure 1. Although milestones are neatly described on a timeline, development is anything but linear – milestones only offer a broad guide for the expected 'typical' development; even for an individual child the development does not progress in a steady and predictable manner in any one *domain*, or at the same rate across all the domains. Some adverse environmental situations, e.g. prolonged hospitalisation or acrimonious separation of parents, may result in plateauing or apparent regression of development.

A stage-like progression has been described for many aspects of development. However, many children show abilities that straddle the stages, skip some stages or do not fit neatly into any particular stage. The methodology of gathering of developmental information, such as frequency of observations (weekly or monthly) and taking a binary view (presence/absence) for gathering information, may contribute to a stage-like appearance of developmental progression even though the actual trajectory may be more continuous and intricate (Adolph and Berger 2006).

> *From Birth to Five Years – Practical Developmental Examination*
>
> ■ Influences on development
>
> ■ Risk and protective factors

Motor development

Achieving stability, balance and independent mobility has a significant role in children becoming active explorers of the world. Neurological maturation provides an important basis for this change, but a number of other factors are now considered to play an important role in creating the flexible and varied course of motor development. Cognitive factors such as perceptual development are closely and reciprocally linked with progress in gross and fine motor skills, known as the action–perception cycle: the physical and social world motivates the infant to interact; the feedback from these interactions in turn facilitates the control of posture and movements. Children adapt and modify their movements and actions according to their growing bodies, changing cognition and skill levels (Adolph and Berger 2006). Their brain, body and experiences make a continually self-organising dynamic system resulting in the progression of skills (Thelen 1995) (see Figure 2).

Experience: action-perception cycle

Children perceive possibilities for action and learn from experience. Their perception of self and the environment changes with experience and learning.

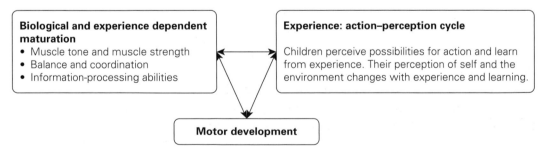

Figure 2 *The continually adaptive dynamic system of motor development.*

The outline sequence of motor development encompasses changes in tone, balance, strength, movement differentiation and coordination leading to the learning of precise skills, with experience playing an increasingly significant role through this progress (Table 2).

Table 2 An outline sequence of motor development (ages serve only as a guide, with much variability and overlap).

Birth–4 months	Primitive reflexes
4 months–1 year	Improving muscle tone – reducing flexor and increasing extensor tone Improving balance and coordination Movements become differentiated and functional
1–2 years	Improving power and stability Better differentiated and more precise movements
3–5+	Improving efficiency in skills, e.g. running, jumping, catching, throwing Applying motor skills for sports and work

Balance and posture

Good balance and a stable postural base are essential for successful action – looking around, handling objects or for mobility. For attaining and maintaining balance and stability we rely on sensory feedback from multiple sources, e.g. our joints (proprioceptive), the position of our head (vestibular) and vision. For the developing infant, the task is harder as the postural base changes during each milestone of motor development – lying, sitting, crawling, cruising and independent walking. The key aspects of postural control for the main postural milestones are described below.

Static posture

For clinical purposes, there is an apparent *cephalocaudal progression* of infants' postural control – first in the muscles of the neck, then in the trunk and finally in the legs (Table 3). Head control is the beginning of the postural control process. Early in infancy the *head righting reflex* maintains the vertical position of the head irrespective of the body position. Once the trunk is stabilised, initially with support and later independently, infants can move their head around and achieve better eye–head–hand coordination.

Table 3 Development of static posture.

			Mean age (range) (in months)
Head control	Supine	Turns head sideways to track objects	1
	Supine	Lifts head up	5
	Pull to sit	Slight head lag	4
	Sitting	Holds head steady	3 (3–4)
	Prone	Lifts head up fully (30–45°)	3
Trunk posture	Sitting	Balanced with straight spine	7 (5–9)
Limbs: range of movements	Arms	Full extension	2
	Legs	popliteal angle: 90°/110°/150°	2/5/9
Hand posture	Supine	Hands mostly open	2 (1–3)

Based on: Frankenburg *et al.* (1975), Piek (2006), Amiel-Tison and Grenier (1986).

Prone posture

In a prone position, infants can lift their heads up by 5–10 weeks of age, and by 3 months they have sufficient control to prop themselves up on their forearms. By 5 months, infants can shift their weight from one arm to the other, thereby freeing their hands to reach for and manipulate toys. By 7–9 months infants can push themselves back, from being on hands and knees, into sitting position and can move from sitting into kneeling or crawling without any intermediate belly flop (Adolph *et al.* 1998).

Sitting

Gradually improving muscle strength and coordination in the neck, trunk and leg muscles enables the infant to sit independently. At 3–4 months old, infants tend to flop forward on their outstretched legs. At approximately 5 months, they sit in a 'tripod' position and prop themselves on their arms with their hands resting on the floor between their outstretched legs. Even as they sit independently at 6 months, they tend to lose balance if they turn to their side. Better trunk and hip control at 7 months gives them the required balance to reach out with their hands to explore. By 8–9 months they can move in and out of sitting position to kneel and crawl – and they are off to explore!

Standing

Infants need both the leg strength and the balance to stand – they have the strength at 7 months but lack the balance. They compensate for it by leaning against a couch or a table, balancing with their arms. They can pull themselves to stand against the furniture by 9 months, first on their toes and then on the flat of their feet. Standing up independently typically comes at the end of the first year.

By 5 months infants have sufficient shoulder strength to turn themselves on to their sides from lying on their tummy, rolling from front to back (prone to supine) by 5–6 months and from back to front by 6–7 months.

Dynamic posture – independent mobility

Rolling

Infants begin belly crawling around 7 months and crawling on hands and knees at 8 months. Not all infants follow the same sequence of sitting, crawling and walking, depending on their *muscle tone* and postural preferences (Table 4). Those who prefer to lie on their tummy or are given 'tummy time', even though they are put on their backs to sleep, have earlier onset ages for sitting, crawling and pulling to stand, presumably because the prone position facilitates muscle strength in the arms and shoulders (Adolph and Berger 2011). Bottom shuffling and creeping/rolling patterns are associated with lower muscle tone, with these infants demonstrating later milestones for sitting and walking.

Crawling

Table 4 Variations in pre-walking development.

Sequence variations	Sit	Crawl	Walk
	Mean/97% (months)	Mean/97% (months)	Mean/97% (months)
Crawl **83%**	7/9	9/13	13/18
Stand and walk **6%**	7/11		11/14
Bottom shuffle **9%**	12/15		17/28
Creep/roll **1%**	9/12	12/17	18/27

Adapted from Robson (1984).

Walking	In order to walk infants have to achieve dynamic balance as their bodies become less stable, because of the smaller base on their feet and higher centre of gravity. They also require sufficient muscle power, particularly in their extensor muscles, to balance the effects of flexors, and gradually change the leg muscle activation from simultaneous co-activation of antagonistic muscles to reciprocal activation. When infants have sufficient strength to hold part of their body weight on one leg, they begin to 'cruise' along furniture by moving sideways, lifting the legs and arms one at a time. As they move forwards, with parents holding their hands, their bodies are tilted 45° forward or backward.

To walk independently sufficient muscle strength and balance control are needed to hold the body on one leg while the other leg swings forward. For the first few months of walking, children have a broad-based *gait*, their feet point in or out and they strike the ground with their toes or the whole foot, with the appearance of 'falling' into each step. After 4–6 months of walking experience the base becomes narrower and steps became longer; their feet contact the floor with a heel–toe progression and arms swing reciprocally with legs. Practice is an important developmental factor for helping infants to strengthen their muscles and improve their balance (Adolph *et al.* 2003).

Up and down stairs	Sometime around the first birthday, most infants develop a love of climbing up and down stars. Crawling up is easier than going down and infants can crawl up a step or two shortly after they can crawl on flat ground. Walking up is harder, achieved not until several weeks after independent walking, initially holding onto the wall or turning sideways to hold a banister with both hands. Walking up stairs without holding a support is achieved at about 30–36 months, and walking down stairs between 3 and 4 years of age.
Spontaneous stereotyped and repetitive movements	Healthy infants spend about 5 per cent of their waking time making apparently stereotyped cyclical movements with arms, hands, legs, trunk and tongue. Most of these movements reach a peak between 4 and 7 months and decline by the end of the first year. Persistence of these movements beyond 18 months of age and

presence of excessive repetitive movements at any age may be an indicator of neuro-developmental abnormalities.

Infants typically acquire new motor skills in a supportive social context (Tamis-LeMonda and Adolph 2005). Caregivers encourage with words, facial expressions, manual gestures, the lure of toys and body position. Walking is often scaffolded by offering a finger to hold onto for support. Some cultures encourage new skills verbally. Others 'train' infants, for example, by propping 3–4 month olds in a special hole in the ground to promote sitting and jumping infants up and down to promote walking (Keller 2003). As a consequence of the variation in child-rearing practices, infants acquire their sitting, crawling, walking and stair-climbing at different rates – at later ages for children with fewer opportunities and less practice (Adolph and Berger 2011).

Cultural variations

Clinicians need to be aware that variations of the norm are common in development. Children who show variations in timing or sequences of development continue to develop normally, and maintaining normal sequences is not a guarantee for appropriate development, e.g. children with mild but significant neurological damage may achieve crawling and walking within the normal range but may have a qualitatively different way of crawling or walking, associated movements or abnormal protective reflexes.

Variations and normative development

> *From Birth to Five Years – Practical Developmental Examination*
> Making sense of findings

All aspects of children's development benefit from opportunities and encouragement to explore. Most children do not need any special considerations for their motor development. Children with impaired neurological maturation benefit from enhanced opportunities, instructions and encouragement, and suitable guidance from a physiotherapist should be obtained. Developmentally appropriate, organised physical activities help children improve in their skills and their general strength, agility and motivation.

Supporting motor development

Amiel-Tison, A. and Grenier, A (1986) *Neurological Assessment during the First Year of Life*. Oxford: Oxford University Press.
Galluhe, D. I. and Ozmum, J. C. (2006) *Understanding Motor Development*. London: McGraw-Hill.

Further reading

Heywood, K. M. and Getchell, N. (2009) *Life Span Motor Development*, 5th edn. Champaign, IL: Human Kinetics.

Piek, J. P. (2006) *Infant Motor Development*. Champaign, IL: Human Kinetics.

Sudgen, D. A. and Wade, M. G. (2013) *Typical and Atypical Motor Development*. London: Wiley.

Fine motor, perceptual and non-verbal cognitive development

Children change from reacting to sensations and making random and uncoordinated movements to perceiving and acting in a planned and coordinated manner. In contrast to movements, actions imply intentionality and goals. For actions to be meaningful, perceptual information and motor abilities need to be complemented by cognitive abilities of understanding, memory, planning and organisation. This coming together of perceptual, motor and cognitive abilities enables children to reach, pick up and play with toys, catch, throw and kick balls and manage day-to-day activities such as using a spoon and fork, dressing and undressing, and learning to write. Development in multiple components of motor and cognitive domains and their ongoing integration contribute to this progress (Figure 3).

From Birth to Five Years – Practical Developmental Examination

Fine motor and non-verbal cognitive development

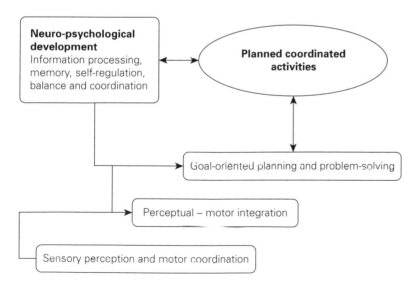

Figure 3 Fine motor and non-verbal cognitive development.

From sensation to perception and action

Children gain information about the world through various sensations: vision, hearing, touch, taste, smell and sensation of movement (kinaesthetic). Sensations become perception when they are connected with stored information and take on meaning to guide thinking and action. Any action generates more information which further guides thinking and action, forming an action–perception loop. Every movement is accompanied by *perceptual feedback*, and many types of visual, tactile, vestibular and proprioceptive information do not exist without movement.

Infants' exploration of the physical and social world

Starting soon after birth infants begin to explore the world through looking, hearing, touching and mouthing. Improvements in the postural balance of head and trunk, eyes–head–hand coordination (first, eyes move with the head to follow an object and, later, hands, eyes and head move together to look at the object held in hand/s) and better control of hand movements combines with improving depth perception to enable infants to reach out and grasp objects. Developing cognitive abilities, e.g. *permanence of object*, means–end relationship, mental representation of objects and the ability to remember and rotate images mentally enables them to search and find, copy and create shapes, models and activities (Figure 4). Fine motor activities thus elicit a combination of progress in motor coordination and non-verbal cognitive abilities.

Finding objects

Infants begin to make sense of object unity (that visible parts of objects are connected) from 3 months and look for partially hidden objects by 6 months. However, it is not until about 9 months that they begin to retrieve completely covered objects (*permanence of object*). By about 12 months they can mentally track an object's hidden movement, so that when a moving toy goes under a table, they anticipate that it will come out at the other end.

Reaching

The development of reaching and grasping is an exemplar of the coming together of progression in balance, strength, coordination, perceptual information about the size and location of the object, intention and *cognition*. Reaching requires stabilising of the body, first achieved in supine and supported sitting, then in independent sitting. In supine and supported sitting infants reach, initially bimanually (4–5 months), and then with just one arm (6 months); by 7 months infants sitting independently reach with one arm in all directions. They now use visual depth perception and improved balance to adjust their posture as they reach out.

Infants can close their fingers against their palms for a palmar grasp by 6 months, tip of index finger against thumb for a pincer grasp by 9 months and have a mature fingertip grasp by 12 months. Improved planning abilities complement motor skills and by 8–9 months of age infants adjust their hands according to the size of objects prior to grasping. They achieve a dynamic *tripod finger grasp* (flexible thumb, index and middle finger grasp) of a pencil by 3 years (Adolph and Berger 2011).

Grasping

From Birth to Five Years – Practical Developmental Examination

Development of grasp

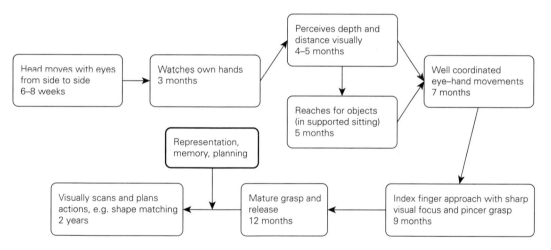

Figure 4 *Visual perception and fine motor development: reaching, exploring and planning.*

After 5–6 months, infants can intentionally release an object, becoming able to transfer it from hand to hand and to rotate it in front of the eyes. However, the mature release of an object, e.g. a 1-inch cube, on a surface is only achieved at about 12 months, enabling the infant to stack two cubes.

Release

Before 4 or 5 months of age infants mainly bring objects to the mouth to explore them orally. By 5 months hand-to-mouth behaviour alternates with holding objects up to the face for visual

Manipulation/ exploration

inspection. At 6–8 months of age, infants relate objects together such as banging on a solid surface to make a noise. By 9 months they begin exploring the surface or a moving part, e.g. the clapper of a bell, with their index finger. The quality of their manipulation of objects has now improved to become more purposeful and they shake or pound more on objects that produce a sound than on objects that do not. Between 12 and 18 months most infants stop bringing objects to their mouths.

Tool use/functional use

From 10 months of age, with improving *cognition* and coordination, infants show *'means–end' concept* by using sticks, attached string or other means to pull objects near. From about 10–12 months they begin to explore objects functionally – using the object for its intended function, e.g. a hairbrush as a brush, initially on self and later on mother/carer and by 18 months on a doll. They have now moved on from simply exploring to using objects as tools (Lockman 2005). At this stage, they still grab a spoon by the bowl-end instead of by the handle. As their planning and coordination improves, by 18–24 months they can adjust their actions, turn the spoon around to hold it properly, and by 24 months use the spoon to get the food out of a bowl. The use of an adult grip of a spoon, between thumb and index finger, however, appears much later – by about 4–5 years of age.

Fitting objects into holes – shape sorting

When children are a little over 12 months old they can just about fit a ball into a circular hole. Until about 22 months of age their attempts to fit other shapes into corresponding apertures only succeed because of their perseverance and acting on feedback – they keep trying different options until they succeed. It is not until they are nearly 2 years old that they can insert a more complicated object, like a cube, into a square aperture (Bayley 1969). From now on, they also start to pre-adjust the orientation of the shape to fit the aperture – a crucial skill needed to succeed. They are now mentally representing the shapes of the aperture and the object and planning their action. By 30 months they can choose one out of two shapes that will match the aperture before they pick up the shape. Most of the errors made from now on are more likely to be due to response inhibition, i.e. an inability to stop themselves picking up the wrong shape, rather than a perceptual-motor ability (Omkloo 2007).

Putting one cube/block on top of another begins at about 12 months, and higher 'towers' are built with improving coordination and planning over the next year or so. Horizontal alignment – making a row of cubes – starts at about 18 months (Stiles and Stern 2001). It is not until 3–4 years that children regularly build both vertical and horizontal components within a single spatial construction (Stiles-Davis 1988). At 24 months, children rely on a simple repetitive process in which one type of relation is used exclusively. This strategy limits constructions to simple stacks or lines. By 36 months, children can use more than one relation but typically generate them in sequence. It is not until 48 months that children produce multi-component constructions and show considerable flexibility, shifting back and forth between different components, in how they generate and integrate different parts of the construction (Stiles-Davis 1988).

Block constructions – spontaneous play or copying

BOX 3 Handedness

Stable handedness, apparent in drawing and constructional play, appears gradually from 2 to 4 years. A child showing strong preference for using only one hand before the age of 18 months, or ignoring the use of one hand at any age, may indicate the presence of neurological abnormality.

Around 10 per cent of people are left-handed. They have to make more adjustments in day-to-day life as almost everything is designed for use by right-handed people. However, a child's *functional difficulties* should not be simply attributed to handedness without careful evaluation.

Continuing progress in perceptual-motor coordination

Gradual improvements occur in finger perceptual discrimination, e.g. finger-to-finger or thumb–finger opposition tasks, and by the age of 4–5 years nearly all children can do this task if demonstrated. By now, they are able to make movements that cross the body midline with ease. From the fourth year onward, children begin to integrate their perceptual, motor and verbal abilities. They are able to have a conversation while doing different activities such as using a knife and fork. They gradually become interested in using the fine motor skills for art and craft activities with increasing sophistication.

From random to planned movements

Motor planning refers to the ability to chain together a series of actions into a purposeful action in an efficient way. Children with difficulties of planning or organising of movements may well understand what is required from a task and have the muscle strength and movements to do the individual components of the task and yet be unable, or find it difficult, to carry out the full sequence, and simple daily tasks such as tying shoelaces can be confusing. Such problems with motor planning may indicate developmental coordination disorder or dyspraxia.

> **BOX 4** Handwriting
>
> Though 3-year-old children begin to copy letters, they place them randomly on the paper. By 5 years they can print their first name with a stable baseline. About half of 5 and 6 year olds write letters wrong way around in 'mirror writing', and a few, about 10 per cent, still do this at age 7 years. Handwriting becomes better organised at 6–9 years of age.

Children's drawings

Children's drawings reflect their fine motor skills, perceptual awareness of the world around them and their representational skills. Initial drawing skills progress from making random marks on paper by 12–15 months, a vigorous to-and-fro scribble by 15–18 months to making circular scribble by the age of 24 months. By 30 months, more intentional circular scribble or immature circles emerge. Toddlers often vocalise while scribbling, as if they were giving a running commentary. By the age of 4, more angles are seen in children's drawings, and they are able to copy a cross and, by 4½ years, a square. At the age of 5 years, children make a clear and accurate oblique cross, the lines become straighter, and angles become sharper. The ability to copy geometric forms, particularly the oblique cross, is seen as an indication of writing readiness in the young child, as it requires crossing the body midline. Towards the end of the fifth year, children are beginning to make three-dimensional representations in their drawings, such as drawing the base of a cylinder.

At around 3–4 years of age, children begin to draw pictures with recognisable features – the most common subject being a human figure. In general, children first draw circles with marks in or around them, proceed to draw arms and then legs projecting directly from the circle by 3 years, then add another circle as a body and more parts at about 4½ years, and the limbs are drawn in two dimensions or width by the age of 5½–6 years.

Drawing human figures

Two- to 3-year-old children normally curl their hands up while running or trying to walk on their heels or toes and move their tongue in and out while drawing or cutting. Most of these associated movements gradually disappear by the age of 7 years, though increasing the difficulty or the stress of the task makes some associated movements appear even in adults. Persistence of these movements or when these movements in some way create difficulty in carrying out age-expected functional tasks would require further assessment.

Associated movements

Children acquire new skills in a supportive social environment. Parents and teachers can help the child by acknowledging the child's difficulty and by applying some general methods to improve the child's functional performance.

Supporting fine motor development

■ Give simple step-by-step instructions for the task.

■ Demonstrate or model activities.

- Model the activity by verbalising steps aloud.

- Allow time for practice.

- Set up a variety of activities.

- Use pictures or written lists to organise activities.

- Reorganise and label things to make them easy for the child to find.

- Consider changing physical environment such as using Velcro, thicker pencils, stable paper pads and adjusting the height of chair/desk.

Further reading

Cermak, S. A. and Larkin, D. (2002) *Developmental Coordination Disorder.* Albany, NY: Delmar Thomson Learning.

Cratty, J. B. (1986) *Perceptual and Motor Development in Infants and Children*, 3rd edn. Englewood Cliffs, NJ: Prentice Hall.

Sudgen, D. and Chambers, M. (2005) *Children with Developmental Coordination Disorder.* London: Whurr Publishers.

Speech, language and communication

Typically developing children are highly competent communicators well before the appearance of recognisable spoken words. By the end of the first year, children can attract and direct an adult's attention, indicate a range of emotions, make clear requests and even make comments or ask questions using a range of non-verbal communication strategies.

Language is a cognitive process that develops in a social context, i.e. it is acquired through interaction with caring and responsive adults rather than through formal instructions. Learning and use of language are influenced by the interaction of biological, cognitive, psycho-social and environmental factors (Figure 5).

Descriptions of children's expressive language are usually given in terms of the different functional aspects: these reflect cognitive, social and motor skills (Table 5).

From Birth to Five Years – Practical Developmental Examination

Speech, language and communication

Learning to communicate

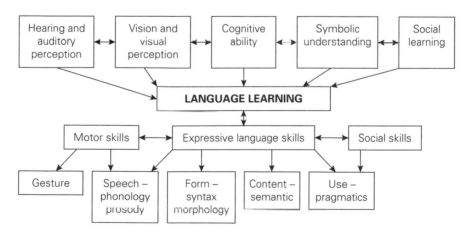

Figure 5 *Factors influencing language learning.*

Table 5 Functional aspects of language.

Speech	Production of sounds
Phonology	The system of consonants and vowels that make up a language
Syntax/grammar	Rules that govern the way that words, and parts of words, combine in phrases and sentences
Morphology	The changes made at word level to convey specific meanings
Semantics	The meaning of sentences, words and parts of words
Pragmatics	How language and non-verbal communication are used in social situations
Prosody	The rhythm (stress) and music (intonation) of speech
Receptive skills	Understanding of language
Expressive skills	Using speech and language to communicate

Theories of language development

As with other aspects of development, there is considerable variation in the age at which children reach specific milestones, but there are similarities in the overall sequence of stages, even across languages. There may be differences in rates of acquisition and in learning styles, and dissociations between components may occur, e.g. some children may be slow to master the sound system of the language whilst achieving typical grammatical milestones.

BOX 5 Bilingualism

On a world scale, monolingualism is unusual. Bilingualism, i.e. 'the knowledge and or use of two or more language codes ... regardless of the relative proficiency of the languages understood or used' (RCSLT 2003), does not result in communication disorders. The limited research available suggests the same proportion of bilingual and monolingual children will have speech and language disorders, and that any difficulties would occur in both languages and would be of a similar type, but that the errors made by the child may be language-specific (Holm *et al.* 2005).

Assessment of the communication skills of bilingual children and intervention for those with speech/language disorders is problematic due to limited knowledge about bilingual language development, a shortage of bilingual professionals and differing cultural views of language development and disorders. A thorough case history may provide some insight into parents' views about the presenting difficulties.

BOX 6 Joint attention

The development of joint attention is a key stage in learning to communicate. The attentional focus of the young infant is the face of a responsive adult or older child. At around 5 months external objects and events become a main interest before, at around 9 months, interactions include another person to become triadic (infant–object–other) and form a shared focus on objects or events (Bruner 1983). Index-finger pointing becomes established just before the first birthday. The ability to follow an adult's eyes/finger pointing, and to direct another's attention to things of interest allows a child to learn the connections between language heard and the objects/events/concepts it represents (mapping). Failure to develop joint attention and *pretend play* behaviours by 18 months has been shown to be highly correlated with childhood autism. Whilst not diagnostic, delayed skills in this area may indicate the need for further neuro-developmental assessment (Baird *et al.* 2000).

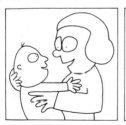 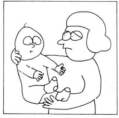 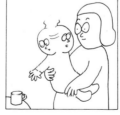 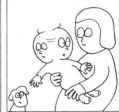

attention to people   *attention to things*   *requesting*   *commenting*

BOX 7 Key stages in language understanding

The ability to interpret the meaning of spoken, and later written, language is built on the child's active mapping of the words and grammatical forms heard in the environment onto the actions, feelings and intentions of self and others. Far from being a simply observational process, or a taught skill, the development of understanding is both a cognitive and a social process. It requires good-quality linguistic input (in whatever language is used in the environment) and caregivers who make the meanings of language clear through their interaction with the child.

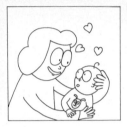

0–3 months
Focuses on a speaker's face

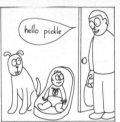

3–6 months
Turns to familiar voices

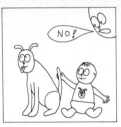

6–9 months
Pauses in response to 'no!'

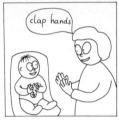

9–12 months
Follows commands in context

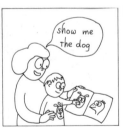

12–18 months
Points to pictures in familiar books

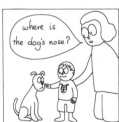

18–24 months
Follows two-part commands

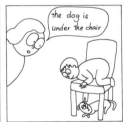

2–4 years
Understands sentences of increasing complexity, including concept words

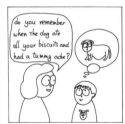

4–6 years
Understands talk about past and future events

BOX 8 Key stages in expressive speech and language development

In parallel with the development of language understanding, infants progress from experimenting with sounds, to specific patterns of sounds that make up recognisable words, and then combining sequences of words, according to language-specific rules, in order to convey increasingly precise meanings. Initially caregivers are required to infer intended meanings from single words or simple word combinations, with meaning becoming less ambiguous as a range of grammatical forms are mastered in the third and fourth years.

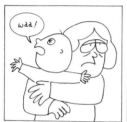

0–2 months
Discomfort cries

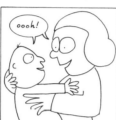

2–4 months
Pleasure sounds

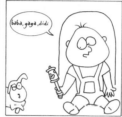

4–9 months
Babbling

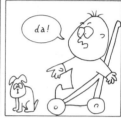

9–12 months
Vocalisations with meaning

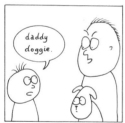

12–15 months
First words

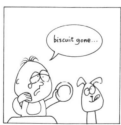

18–30 months
Two-word phrases

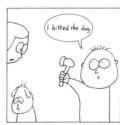

2½–4 years
Developing syntax

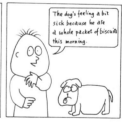

4–6 years
Adult syntax

Language for learning

Children utilise their communication skills in the expression of needs and wants, to share information and interests, for the purposes of social closeness and for social etiquette. In addition, effective oral-language skills provide the basis for subsequent literacy and numeracy development. The impact of a communication delay or disability on reading and spelling is well recognised and one of the motivations for providing advice and support for parents in the early stage of development.

It has been estimated that up to 50 per cent of children in the UK arrive at school lacking the communication skills necessary for an effective start to learning, most commonly in regions where there is socio-economic disadvantage (Locke *et al.* 2002). This delay is often specific to language, with the children having motor, visual perceptual and general cognitive skills comparable to the general population. Most of these children will have transient difficulties and are likely to catch up with their peers given appropriate support. Ten per cent of children can be described as having a communication disability (1.2 million in the UK), with 6 per cent having a specific and persistent communication disability (I CAN 2006).

Supporting language and communication development

Strategies to support communication

Parents and other caregivers have a fundamental role in supporting communication development. General advice would be directed at enhancing the skills that most parents bring to interaction with the child.

- In the early months, talk to the baby, even when the baby is not talking back, particularly during care routines and play.

- Respond to the baby's actions as if they have meaning.

- Minimise background noise so babies can listen to speech.

- Simplify speech: use short sentences, emphasise keywords, use gestures and leave pauses for the child to contribute.

- Follow the child's attention and talk about what he/she is looking at for a short period on a daily basis.

- Use everyday activities for language learning, e.g. putting away the shopping, sorting the laundry, etc.

- Establish a daily routine of joint picture-book reading – talk about the pictures, rather than simply asking 'Where's the. . .?' or 'What's that?' questions.

- Elaborate on what the child has said, e.g. add descriptions, explain causes and effects, talk about people's emotions and motivations, etc.

All of these skills are used intuitively by parents and others who spend large amounts of time with young children. However, parents show variation in their levels of responsiveness and skill. Factors such as maternal depression, family stress and limited contact between children and parents may result in children receiving impoverished language input and are therefore important to explore during assessment.

Further reading

Buckley, B. (2003) *Children's Communication Skills: From Birth to Five Years*. London: Routledge.

Dockrell, J. and Messer, D. (1999) *Children's Language and Communication Difficulties: Understanding, Identification and Intervention*. London: Cassell.

Hoff, E. and Shatz, M. (2007) *Blackwell Handbook of Language Development*. Chichester: Wiley-Blackwell.

Saxton, M. (2010) *Child Language: Acquisition and Development*. London: Sage.

Winkler, E. (2012) *Understanding Language: A Basic Course in Linguistics*, 2nd edn. London: Continuum.

Social behaviour and play

From Birth to Five Years – Practical Developmental Examination

Social behaviour and play

Social cognition: Development of social understanding

Babies are born into a complex social world. Through active participation in interactions with people more skilled than themselves – adults and children, familiar and unfamiliar – children develop an understanding of the actions, desires, feelings, intentions and beliefs of others. This enables them to form and maintain relationships and to learn the conventions of behaviour within the society. From 2 months of age, parents and infants are able to hold each other's attention and engage in intricate, mutually regulated interchanges, primary intersubjectivity (Trevarthen and Aitken 2001). This 'dance' of social communication is the beginning of the infant's learning of social behaviour (see Table 6).

Play

Children's play with objects, carers and peers evolves with age. This progression is closely tied to cognitive, symbolic and social development (Table 7). Consequently, observation of children's play is a rich source of information about developmental abilities.

Pretend play (also described as symbolic, make-believe or imaginary play) is perhaps the most fascinating aspect of child development. It starts around 12 months with a functional use of objects, largely in a scripted and imitative manner, first on self and then on others. By the age of 4–5 years, children make the most creative use of language and objects to act out a fantastic world of imagination which they share with their peers and carers.

Table 6 Key stages in social development.

	Child	Carer's role
0–6 weeks	■ Preference for attending to people ■ Recognition of mother's voice ■ Intent regard of faces	■ Treating infant as a communicating being ■ Sympathetic and expressive behaviour that holds the infant's attention
6–8 weeks	■ Smiling emerges ■ Imitation of facial expressions	■ Sustained interaction sequences ■ Recognising the need for pauses and withdrawal to avoid over-excitement
3 months	■ Smiling and other facial expressions synchronised with those of caregivers	■ Developing social routines
5 months	■ Growing interest in objects ■ Some refusal to look at parents	■ Developing games with objects in order to maintain interaction
9 months	■ Using referential gaze to direct parent's attention to objects	■ Following the infant's focus of attention
10 months	■ Wary of strangers	■ Offering reassurance – remaining close by modelling friendly behaviour
1–2 years	■ Understands that others' acts are intentional ■ Reactions to novel situations largely dependent on that of caregiver (*social referencing*) ■ Development of teasing – anticipating parent's reaction to forbidden actions ■ Protest and tantrums – limit testing	■ Modelling appropriate social behaviour ■ Joint book reading – focusing on objects and actions ■ Direct coaching – please, thank you, sorry, etc. ■ Setting standards and teaching permitted/forbidden behaviour
2–3 years	■ Understands that others act on their desires and beliefs ■ Understanding of responsibility – leading to denial of transgressions ■ Asking 'what' and 'where' questions ■ Captivated by stories – focus shifts from actions of characters to feelings	■ Commenting and making suggestions during play ■ Consistency in limit setting ■ Direct coaching in polite behaviour ■ Joint book reading – focusing on mental states
3–4 years	■ Breadth of interest in social world ■ Asking 'why' questions ■ Talk about inner states and rules – what is good, bad, naughty, allowed, etc. ■ Able to adopt emotional states within pretend play	■ Providing information and explanations of the actions of people in social situations and stories
4–5 years	■ Understands that others may be acting on a *false belief* ■ Growing understanding of rules ■ Increasing understanding of the links between people's mental state and actions – theory of mind (Box 9)	■ Supervision of games and play with peers ■ Supporting social understanding

Table 7 Cognitive and social dimensions of play.

	Cognitive dimension	Social dimension
From 6 to 8 weeks	**Early parent–child social play** ■ Intent looking ■ Imitation of facial expressions ■ Vocalisations ■ Actions become more purposeful through contingent responses	■ Shared enjoyment ■ Mutual reciprocal responsiveness in actions, e.g. smiling, touching ■ From about 6 months, rough and tumble play becomes a major source of shared fun
From 5 months	**Object (e.g. toys) exploration and manipulation** ■ Visual regard and eye–hand coordination ■ Exploration of objects – touching, banging, mouthing ■ Targeted actions – pressing buttons, pulling strings – to obtain specific effects (9 months)	■ Toys become the focus of shared attention with carers ■ Infant initiates by holding up or offering toys in order to enlist adult in interaction ■ Happy responsiveness to exciting social interactions, e.g. peek-a-boo is well established by 9 months
From 10 to 12 months	**Functional play** ■ Use of common objects, e.g. using a hairbrush, putting on hat, 'talking' on phone	■ Looks for approval and encouragement and, following a positive response, uses common objects on carers
From 12 to 21 months	**Pretend play – *simple imitative pretence*** ■ Using miniature toys functionally on self (from 12 months) ■ Using toys functionally on the parent/carer (15–18 months) and on a doll (18–21 months); initially using simple toys, e.g. cup, spoon and, later, other objects, e.g. blanket, bottle	■ Initial self-directed play becomes other-directed from 18 to 21 months, inviting interaction from carers ■ Most of these actions are deferred imitations of commonly observed activities and are often initiated or reinforced by carers
From 24 months	**Pretend play – *sequential imitative pretence*** ■ Integrates two- or three-step actions, e.g. feeds the doll and covers with a blanket ■ Begins to play with substitution objects, e.g. can use something that is not much like a cup to feed the doll	■ Play remains a reproduction of commonly observed activities, which are encouraged by carers ■ Adults join in the play with some turn taking, e.g. for 'tea and snack' ■ Plays alongside other children, playing with similar toys and watching others

	Cognitive dimension	Social dimension
2–2½ years	**Pretend play – *giving 'life' or agency to toys***	
	■ Gives *agency* to toys, e.g. makes a doll 'say' something or do something (feed another doll) ■ Able to use two or more substitutions, e.g. a rolled-up towel as a doll and a crayon as a bottle	■ Most play sequences at this stage still appear somewhat 'scripted' and simulations of observed activities
3–4 years	**Pretend play – *awareness of pretence***	
	■ Children know and say that they are pretending, e.g. 'this towel is my baby' ■ Longer sequences: by age 4 years they can combine four related themes, e.g. feeding, kissing it goodnight, laying in bed and covering with a blanket	■ Approaches and joins with other children, often comments on others' play. Sharing materials but often pursuing own ideas ■ From age 3 years children involve others in 'role play', initially copying observed activities from real life or TV, e.g. doctor/patient, mother/child
4 –5 years	**Pretend play – *using language to share imagination***	
	■ Uses language to frame pretend play, e.g. 'this is my shop' ■ Creation of conventional and fantasy scenarios	■ Shares own belief and plan with peers ■ Negotiates with peers with appreciation of rules ■ The relationship between social pretend and language is dynamic with each influencing the other

Sources: Pellegrini (2009), Cohen (2006), Curry and Arnaud (1984), Belsky and Most (1981), McCune-Nicolich (1981).

Development of friendships

The development of children's friendships provides a vehicle for, and a reflection of, changes in social understanding. From the age of 18 months, children demonstrate a growing awareness of other children and respond in increasingly sophisticated ways, modifying their behaviour in the context of peer interaction (Table 8).

In early childhood, siblings often show a mix of concern and hostility towards one another. Teasing of parents and older siblings emerges from around 15 months, with children engaging in increasingly elaborate actions to annoy. There is evidence of strong attachments to older siblings from early in the second year. Siblings are generally able to cooperate to some degree in play by 3 years. By 4 years, children have developed the capacity to provide emotional support to distressed younger siblings.

Table 8 Stages in development of friendships.

18 months	Child shows awareness of another child's distress
20 months	Mutual imitation
	Beginning to cooperate with a sibling/peer in order to achieve a goal
2 years	Development of preferences for particular companions
	Cooperating within a shared play theme, e.g. a tea party
2½ years	Able to adopt complementary roles within play scenarios, e.g. doctor/patient, mother/baby
3 years	Awareness of what is pretence, e.g. pretending to be in pain, a hungry baby, etc. Using references to friendship to include and exclude, e.g. 'I'm not your friend today'
	Tendency to label any play companion as a friend, therefore can appear fickle
	Development of 'fighting friends', i.e. reciprocal relationships that include both harmonious play and conflict
	Some children develop imaginary friends
4 years	Children are clear about who their friends are and will differentiate between friends and other peers
	Development of sophisticated sharing of a pretend world. Play includes sustained adventures, often including favourite characters from books or films, or everyday events
	Fantasy play with strong emotional components such as fear, abandonment, bravery
	Alternative types of reciprocal play include sharing physical activities (chasing, playing football or skipping) or shared mischief
5 years	Increasing understanding of the needs, feelings and wishes of friends
	Bargaining, compromise and reconciliation
	Able to talk about what makes someone a friend

BOX 9 Theory of Mind

Theory of Mind refers to a person's capacity to attribute feelings, thoughts and beliefs to others, and to the understanding that actions are governed by those feelings, thoughts and beliefs. The development of social cognition involves looking beyond external behaviours to make inferences regarding desires, intentions and motivations.

As an area of ability that is considered crucial in social interaction and communication there has been extensive research into the Theory of Mind capabilities of individuals with autistic spectrum disorders, giving rise to the concept of 'mind blindness'. Theory of Mind tasks involve creating social scenarios and asking children questions about what characters have seen, what they are thinking and what they are likely to do. Associations have been established between the ability to solve Theory of Mind tasks, pretend play, joint attention and language skills.

Parents support the development of their children's awareness of mental states through conversation about emotions, thoughts and beliefs of others, making the mental states of others explicit, and so leading to a coherent Theory of Mind. These conversations occur in the contexts of everyday social situations, play, watching films and television programmes, and in shared book reading.

Supporting social behaviour and play

Parents, caregivers and early years professionals play a crucial role in supporting a child's social development. The emphasis should be on creating opportunities rather than direct teaching of skills.

- Creating distraction-free time for interaction with infants.

- Creating opportunities for social play: action songs, turn-taking games, joint interactive play, and joint book-reading.

- Valuing children's play.

- Providing age-appropriate play materials.

- Sharing the excitement of children's discoveries and achievements.

Theory of Mind

- Supporting the development of peer relationships: taking turns, sharing, making requests, passing toys, etc.

- Direct coaching in polite behaviour.

- Consistent management of behaviour, with clear boundaries and consequences.

Further reading

Carpendale, J. and Lewis, C. (2006) *How Children Develop Social Understanding*. Oxford: Blackwell.

Cohen, D. (2006) *The Development of Play*, 3rd edn. London: Routledge.

Dunn, J. (2003) *Children's Close Relationships: Beyond Attachment*. Oxford: Blackwell.

Dunn, J. (2004) *Children's Friendships: The Beginnings of Intimacy*. Oxford: Blackwell.

Harris, P. L. (2000) *The Work of the Imagination*. Oxford: Blackwell.

Nelson, K. (2007) *Young Minds in Social World: Experience, Meaning and Memory*. Cambridge, MA: Harvard University Press.

Pellegrini, A. D. (2009) *The Role of Play in Human Development*. Oxford: Oxford University Press.

Sheridan, M. (2011) *Play in Early Childhood: From Birth to Six Years*, 3rd edn, rev. by J. Howard and D. Alderson. London: Routledge.

Early literacy development

One of the key tasks for childhood is to learn to read and write. Literacy skills are the foundations for further educational attainment and, although many children may not be able to read before they start school, the skills underpinning literacy are acquired from birth to 5 years.

At age 5, there will be considerable variation in literacy skills: some children may be able to recognise a selection of written words and make an attempt to write their own name, while others will be at the stage of recognising familiar logos. Most will recognise that print has meaning. Being sung to, read to and engaged in other literacy-related activities by caregivers will have contributed to literacy readiness.

Before learning to read and spell, children will have developed the speech-processing skills required for understanding and producing intelligible spoken language. Language development itself can be enhanced through early literacy experiences. In particular, being actively engaged in shared book reading with a supportive adult has a powerful influence on language acquisition. Strategies such as expanding on what the child says and asking open-ended questions (rather than simply asking the child to name the pictures) are associated with enhanced language growth in toddlers and pre-schoolers. A positive relationship exists between the number of picture books in the home, and children's receptive and expressive skills.

Aspects of the home learning environment such as being read to, visiting libraries, singing nursery rhymes and other children's songs, playing with letters and numbers, and having attention drawn to letters and sounds have all been shown to have a positive impact on children's school readiness and attainments at least in the early school years. Parallel developments across the multiples domains all contribute to the acquisition of early literacy skills (Figure 6).

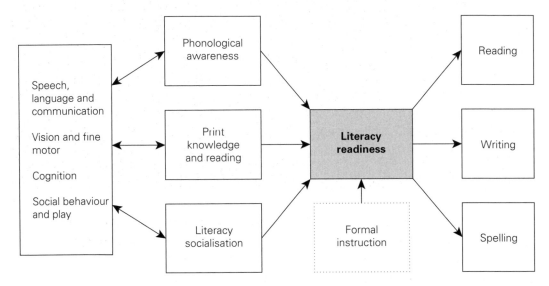

Figure 6 *Factors contributing to literacy readiness.*

Literacy socialisation

By being read to from infancy children learn to associate books with enjoyment and social closeness. Learning how books work, including holding the book the right way up, turning pages, orienting the book so that listeners can see the pictures, the relationship of pictures and text, and following print with an index finger from left to right, are all acquired through repeated modelling and prompting. From around 2 years of age children learn that turning the page is necessary in order to move on to the next part of the story, and also that turning pages too quickly interrupts the story. Pictures in books provide a joint focus of attention that facilitates language mapping, i.e. matching spoken words to the things they represent. By reading the same book multiple times children also understand that print is stable, i.e. the same words are spoken each time the book is read, even by different people. Indeed, young children often go through a phase of being extremely upset if the reader tries to skip parts of a highly familiar text.

BOX 10 The language of literacy

It is usually in the context of reading, rather than speaking, that children learn the vocabulary used to describe units of language: terms including *words, letters, sounds, sentences, pages, rhymes, poems, stories, reading* and *writing* all develop meaning as a child becomes literate. The language of storytelling conventions such as 'once upon a time . . .', 'let's pretend', 'what do you think happened next' and 'the end' become familiar through both story books and oral storytelling. Literary language, i.e. the language used in books and to tell stories, differs from oral language in syntactic complexity and the use of more precise and abstract vocabulary; for this reason, familiarity with books before formal instruction in learning to read provides children with an advantage at school entry.

Phonological awareness

The early stages of becoming a reader (being able to decode print) involve the development of segmentation skills, i.e. segmenting sentences into words, words into syllables and syllables into sounds/letters. These skills are often referred to as phonological awareness. Exposure to rhymes in the form of lap games, nursery rhymes, poems, songs and books written in rhyme provides children with awareness of word sound patterns, leading to the ability to segment words into syllables. The ability to detect and generate rhymes has been associated with success in learning to read and write. From around 4 years of age children frequently enjoy playing with rhyme, noticing rhymes, substituting alternative rhymes within familiar songs and inventing nonsense rhymes. Segmenting words into syllables, e.g. *to-ma-to,* is also of interest to 4 and 5 year olds. The next stage of phonological awareness would be to identify words with the same beginning sound (alliteration) with children enjoying games of I-spy. Subsequent phonological awareness skills include identifying words with the same final sound, e.g. *dog* and *frog*, splitting words into component sounds, e.g. *d-o-g*, and manipulating sounds within words, e.g. *frog without r makes fog*.

Print knowledge and reading

Between the ages of 2 and 5 years, in parallel to learning about stories and the narrative aspects of books, children will develop knowledge of the characteristics of print, and how these relate to speech. Learning the alphabet song, i.e. a musical recitation of the letters of the alphabet, may be a starting point, although this is not typically associated with print. Alphabet books (of the 'A is for apple, B is for bear. . .' variety) introduce the concept that letter shapes are associated with specific speech sounds. By school entry children may have knowledge of letter *names* and letter *sounds*, although this is typically patchy with areas of confusion. The initial letter of child's own name is commonly the first to be recognised.

Through following adults pointing to print as they read, children learn that clusters of letters, framed by spaces, are words, and may start to recognise the shapes of some words that have been seen repeatedly. Again, it is typically the child's own name that is of sufficient interest and exposure to become the first word a child can 'read'. Children who have had experience of being read to will often 'pretend' to read either to themselves or to toys and younger children, i.e. turning the pages of a book and reciting from memory or describing the pictures.

In addition to books, print in the environment provides functional literacy experience. Signs, notices, shop names reinforce that notion that print is an important source of information. Some children will be persistent in their requests for adults to tell them 'what does that say?' and will delight in their ability to recognise familiar logos, shop names and road signs.

Recognition of whole printed words in books may emerge around 5 years of age, with significant variation due to practice and language skills. Decoding, i.e. being able to identify the correct sounds for printed letters and synthesizing sounds across letters to form words, is often associated with formal education, but some families will have focused on these skills in the fifth year. Decoding is dependent on the child developing the necessary phonological awareness.

Children start to make marks on paper from 15 months of age, with the ability to control a pencil sufficiently to draw lines and 'V' shapes from around 2 years. In the third and fourth years mastery of a dynamic tripod grip and non-verbal perceptual and cognitive development enable children to copy shapes of increasing complexity, including letters. Drawing and writing become distinct activities. By 5 years of age most children will make an attempt to write their name and may attempt to label their drawings using invented spellings, with some recognisable letters. Between five and six spellings for common words are learned, and children start to spell by segmenting words into sounds and writing letters that correspond to those sounds.

The experiences offered to young children will depend on the carer's own attitude to, and confidence in, their literacy skills. Reading and writing are 'secondary codes', i.e. representations of spoken language, and therefore are closely related to knowledge and use of language. Children's language understanding and use of vocabulary at 2 years are strongly associated with performance on entering primary school, therefore strategies to support speech, language and communication will have benefit for later literacy skills (see Speech, language and communication, p. 85 above). Children growing up in non-English-speaking or -reading homes can have rich literacy socialisation experiences through lap games, songs, rhymes, oral stories and books from the home culture.

- The rhythms and repetitive language of songs and rhymes support language learning.

- Reading aloud combines the benefits of speaking, listening and storytelling within a single activity.

- Stories can invite children to anticipate and contribute.

- Talking about pictures in books is as important as reading the text.

- Books can introduce children to vocabulary and situations outside their daily lives.

Writing and spelling

From Birth to Five Years – Practical Developmental Examination

Fine motor and non-verbal cognitive development

Supporting early literacy

- Telling stories about a child's own experiences helps children to learn to express their thoughts and feelings.

- Books can help carers to overcome inhibitions and provide topics for discussion.

Further reading

Hamer, C. (2012) *NCT Research Overview: Parent–Child Communication Is Important from Birth*. http://www.literacytrust.org.uk/assets/0001/3375/Hamer_NCT_research_overview_Parent_child_communication_p15-20_Mar12.pdf (accessed 3 June 2013).
Snowling, M. J. (2002) 'Reading and Other Learning Difficulties', in M. Rutter and E. Taylor (eds), *Child and Adolescent Psychiatry*, 4th edn. Oxford: Blackwell Scientific, pp. 682–96.

Web resources

www.wordsforlife.org.uk
www.literacytrust.org.uk

Self-regulation of emotions and attention

As children develop their language, social and cognitive skills they also get better at paying *attention* to what is relevant, managing their emotions appropriately for the situation and thinking and planning about events and problems. This improvement in self-regulation and organising abilities helps them adapt to the demands of schooling, supports learning, reduces aggression and behaviour problems and helps peer socialisation with their peer group (Figure 7). The development of self-regulation is shaped by a combination of developing pre-frontal cortex in the brain, emotional experiences of parent–child relationship and improvements of language, memory and other cognitive abilities (Garon *et al.* 2008). Self-regulation is a crucial link between children's genetic predisposition, early experience and their functional competence (Thompson *et al.* 2013).

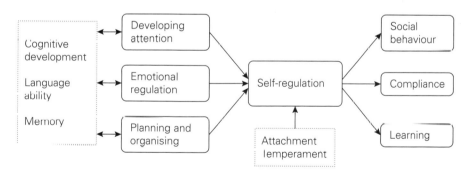

Figure 7 *Self-regulation: underpinning processes and outcomes.*

Regulating emotions does not mean suppressing emotions but expressing emotions effectively and appropriately for safety, **Emotional regulation** getting one's needs met and socialising. Crying loudly secures a carer's attention and has a protective role for an infant; loud expression of anger on not getting his/her own way may be asserting a sense of identity and self-control for a 2 year old. However, by about the age of 3 years children are learning to modulate their displeasure, anger and frustrations, enabling them to work alongside their peer group.

Parental responses help children develop regulation: during infancy parents help children manage their emotions by soothing or distracting them; from about 12 months onwards children begin to 'check back' (*social referencing*) and parents start providing them with social rules and expectations, and sometimes by ignoring children's emotional outbursts parents give a message that a particular emotional response does not get attention. As children improve in their language understanding parents help children manage their emotions by providing reassurance (e.g. 'I know you are sad but you are going to be alright'), alternative meaning of an emotional stimuli (e.g. '– did not mean to upset you, it was an accident') or other alternatives (e.g. 'why don't we make a card to say that you are sorry'). Gradually the control of emotional expression shifts from needing external help to becoming internalised self-regulation and from objects and people to understanding and reasoning (Table 9) (Thompson *et al.* 2013).

Development of attention

Within the first few days of birth infants begin to focus selectively on faces, bright toys or interesting sounds, e.g. mother's voice. This ability to attend, to engage meaningfully and to learn goes through further developments (Table 10) to enable a child to:

a. ignore distractions and pay selective attention to a stimulus or activity;
b. maintain alertness and sustain attention long enough;
c. not perseverate but shift attention to a new and important event; and
d. by the age of 5 years deploy and control attention flexibly to more than one activity at the same time, e.g. do a task while listening to directions (Ruff and Rothbart 1996).

Table 9 Development of emotional and behavioural regulation.

Age group	Emotional and behavioural expression	Regulatory processes
Birth–3 months	Responding to voice and maternal facial expressions. Smiles in response and gives other facial expressions of distress and pleasure. Easily over aroused or distressed.	Responds to soothing voice and close contact from carer. Closes eyes or sucks thumb for self-soothing.
3–6 months	Responds to joyful interactions by smiling and making sounds. Facial expression of anger.	Responds readily to emotions in the face and voice of carers. Comforted by close contact and soothing voice.
7–12 months	Shows wariness of stranger and facial expression of sadness on separation from mother. Shows understanding of daily routines.	'Checks back' with carer and is assured by carer's voice and expressions. Is now able to look away and avoid distressing stimulus.
18 months– 3 years	Shows some secondary emotions such as shame and pride. Uses emotion words from 2 years. Carries out own intentions. Frequent emotional outbursts, 'tantrums'. Verbalises everyday rules: 'mummy said don't put toys in the washing basket'.	Begins to comply with verbal directions and responds to verbal praise and reassurance.
3–4 years	Expresses complex emotions. Able to understand others' emotions. 'Uses' emotions to negotiate. Knows behavioural rules, e.g. 'don't hurt others'.	Able to use some rules, responds to structure and plans to guide behaviour.
4–5 years	Can inhibit an emotion and curb a desire to take the first thing offered – waits to see what else is on offer. Can disengage from one mindset and make a shift to start something new. Talks about right/wrong and understands that some behaviour is inappropriate.	True 'self-regulation' with sophisticated understanding of causes and consequences. Hides and modulates emotions as appropriate to situation.

Sources: Kopp and Wyer (1994), Kopp (1982).

By 2–3 months infants focus their attention more on patterned or complex rather than simple or bright stimuli. At this stage, they have difficulty in disengaging and shifting their attention and carers help them by vocalising and directing. As they get better at

Orienting and exploring

reaching and grasping they seem more interested in objects than in people and can shift attention from one focus to another easily by 6 months, mainly to search for novel and interesting objects.

Table 10 Stages of attention development.

Stage 1: First year	High level of distractibility towards bright and dominant stimuli
Stage 2: Second and third year	Rigid and single-channelled attention on a task of own choice, resistance to input from carers, attention shifts need help from carers
Stage 3: Third and fourth year	Early integrated attention: children can control their own focus of attention – need to look towards the carer to listen
Stage 4: Fifth year	Mature integrated attention: can perform an activity while listening to the carer/teacher giving directions
Stage 5: Fifth year onwards	Flexible and sustained attention based on goals and plans

Based on Cooper *et al.* (1978), Ruff and Rothbart (1996).

Sharing attention

By the end of the first year, infants are less interested in novelty and exploration and more in what others do. They are now good at joint attention, i.e. directing others' attention or following the direction of others' attention to share or respond to others' interest. They also begin to sustain their attention better on what *they plan to do* rather than on simple exploration or novelty – they are now beginning to self-regulate their attention as carers encourage them by praising their efforts.

Alertness and sustained attention

Objects and events looked at with close attention are learnt and remembered better. When children sustain attention they look interested and calm, with decreased body movements and intent facial expression. Motivation, temperament and cognitive ability to generate and carry out longer sequences of activity help to sustain attention. From the age of 2 years onwards children's own goals and plans make their attention less vulnerable to distractions. A major problem characteristic of children with Attention Deficit and Hyperactivity Disorder (ADHD) is difficulty in sustaining the effort necessary to persist at a task and a strong tendency to seek immediate rewards (Ruff and Rothbart 1996: 202).

Parents help to regulate attention of infants and young children by increasing their alertness through supporting their posture, verbally directing attention, demonstrating and pausing, providing structure and playing in a more task-oriented manner. From age 18 months children have a better sense of self and enjoy praise when they get things right. From age 2 to 3 years they begin to inhibit their impulses and act carefully, monitoring their actions themselves. From age 3 years they sometimes use 'private' speech to guide their actions. Between the ages of 3 and 5 years children get better at dealing with conflicting demands on attention. Initially, at age 3 years, they seem to get stuck with one way of dealing with a problem, such as sorting objects based on function or colour. By age 4 they can disengage from one mindset to follow another line of thinking, e.g. stop sorting by colour and switch to sorting by function. They are gradually less reliant on directions from others and can exercise their internal control. Their *working memory* can now hold more information to carry through a task to completion and children become more deliberate in selecting and holding their attention. Attention now becomes a reflection of learning and source for making fewer errors (Berger *et al.* 2007).

Regulating attention

Children's ability to self-regulate their emotions and attention emerge in the context of care-giving relationships (Thompson *et al.* 2013). Parents support the development of self-regulation through:

Supporting the development of self-regulation

- Providing predictable routines, through repeated patterns of asking and praising.

- Modelling behaviour.

- Direct coaching (e.g. asking the child to say sorry or comfort their friend or sibling or encouraging them to take turns).

- Gradually helping children to do things by themselves.

The praise and support that children get from their parents is an important resource for self-regulation. Some children need more support than others and for longer times. It can be a very different challenge for children with different temperaments or for children with a variety of diagnosed disabilities and for their caregivers. Advice may be available from local parenting support groups or child mental health services. There are some general skills and methods that parents can use to help their child's attention and self-regulation:

- Get the child's attention before speaking.

- Get the child to look at you in the eye, even by gently holding their hands and pointing their face towards yours.

- Speak clearly, without shouting.

- Turn off other distractions such as television/radio/music.

- Set up routines.

- Praise and be positive, reward the child for being good.

- Help the child to think before taking an action: set up a stop–think–act routine.

- Encourage children to talk about their feelings and experience after they have done something.

- Use books and stories to talk about emotions.

Further reading

Berger, A., Kofman, O., Livneh, U. and Henik, A. (2007) 'Multidisciplinary Perspective on Attention and the Development of Self-regulation', *Progress in Neurobiology* 82: 256–86.

Ruff, H. A. and Rothbart, M. K. (1996) *Attention in Early Development*. New York: Oxford University Press.

Thompson, R. A., Virmani, E. A., Waters, S. F., Raikes, H. A. and Meyer, S. (2013) 'The Development of Emotional Self-regulation – the Whole and the Sum of Parts', in K. C. Barrett, N. A. Fox, G. A. Morgan, D. A. Fidler and L. A. Daunhauer (eds), *Handbook of Self-regulatory Processes*. New York: Psychology Press, pp. 5–26.

Attachment, temperament and the development of self

Children's interactions with carers are based on mutual love and affection, socialising and play, the need to be cared for and attachment. Attachment refers to the infant's selective and enduring emotional connection with an adult caregiver. Beginning at about 6–7 months of age, infants seek proximity with the primary attachment figure (usually the mother) for security and comfort. Such a sense of security enables the infant to confidently explore the environment in the knowledge that s/he can return to the attachment figure in the face of any threat. The caregiver's sensitivity and motivation in reading the infant's signals, and quality of their responses, form the basis of a two-way relationship between the infant and the carer. Once a selective attachment with a primary caregiver is established children usually form multiple and often simultaneous attachments with other carers, e.g. father, grandparents, aunts and older siblings. Generally two or three such attachments form during childhood, with a hierarchical order of preference. Compared to those with a history of poor attachment relationships, children with a secure and stable attachment history are generally more capable of developing and maintaining successful relationships, better emotional regulation and a more positive sense of self as adults (Thompson 2008).

Attachment behaviour is what children do, when they are stressed or threatened, e.g. on separation from the attachment figure, to seek or maintain proximity, and the way they express their happiness on reunion with them. As expected, with the development of social, cognitive and emotional abilities, these behaviours change (Table 11). Children also show different attachment behaviour depending on the setting and cultural expectations, e.g. in the home they may show low-intensity behaviours such as smiling

ATTACHMENT

Theory of attachment

Development of attachment behaviour

and approaching visitors, while outside or in stressful situations they may show high-intensity behaviours such as wanting to be picked up or staying close to their primary caregivers (Grossman *et al.* 2005). The attachment behaviour in children age 3 years or more becomes more verbal with eye contact or aversion used for proximity or avoidance.

Table 11 Normal development of attachment behaviour and relationships.

	Child	Caregiver
Birth or soon after to 3–4 months	Social interaction emerges with preference for human face and mother's voice, smiling, cooing and excited movements.	Maintains proximity, shows affection and protects. Initiates or sensitively responds to reciprocal interactions involving smiling/touching.
4 months to 7	Begins to show some preference towards one or a few principal caregivers (knows who the main carers are), but generally remains comfortable with any carer.	Caregivers frequently respond to infant's approaches and express joy in interactions; also initiate such interactions for mutual expressions of affection; show understanding of distress and soothe with affection.
7 months to 18 months	Shows selective attachment towards the main carer, usually the mother. Approaches and follows the mother. Shows joy with smile as greeting and distress on separation and wariness towards strangers. Explores freely in mother's presence as a 'secure base', often checking back with her.	The mother anticipates differential attachment and encourages approaches. Initiates or responds to vocalising and gestural communication.
18 months to 2–3 years	Continuing connection with the mother as a 'secure base' for exploration forays. Obtains mother's attention by vocalising, showing anger or crying. Follows the mother and becomes distressed on separation. Uses words to label emotions.	Mother monitors child's explorations for safety and security, provides immediate and appropriate responses to child's 'checking back' and carries the child if required.
3–4 years	Calls and actively searches for the mother on separation, but better able to tolerate separation if other familiar adults are around.	Carers continue to offer close proximity and introduce familiar adults with reassurance.

	Child	Caregiver
	Requires less physical contact with the attachment figure but still seeks brief proximity before returning to exploration/play.	
4 years+	Able to tolerate brief separations with the main carer if the reason is explained and negotiated – understands caregiver's feelings and goals,	Carers listen to the child. Carers explain risks of situations. Carers negotiate by explaining reasons and advantages/risks.
	Intimate interactions are now mainly with eye contact, non-verbal expressions and conversations.	
	Increasingly comfortable spending time in the company of non-familiar peers and adults.	

Source: Marvin and Britner (2008).

Although attachment behaviour may only be expressed by the child under stress, attachment relationships are apparent in other common features of parent–child interactions, e.g. sharing of affection, maintaining proximity and positively resolving any difficulties.

Individual difference in patterns of attachment behaviours

Ainsworth, based on her long observational studies of infants' responses in stressful situations during the Strange Situation Procedure (SSP) (Box 11), described distinct patterns of attachment behaviours (Ainsworth *et al.* 1978).

> **BOX 11** Strange Situation Procedure
>
> The child is observed playing for about 20 minutes while caregivers and strangers enter and leave the room, recreating the flow of the familiar and unfamiliar presences in most children's lives. The situation varies in stressfulness and the child's responses are observed. Four aspects of the child's behaviour are observed:

1. The amount of exploration (e.g. playing with new toys) the child engages in throughout.

2. The child's reactions to the departure of its caregiver.

3. The *stranger wariness* (when the baby is alone with the stranger).

4. The child's reunion behaviour with its caregiver.

These attachment patterns (secure, insecure and disorganised) are not clinical diagnoses and are not an indicator of the strength of attachment. Infants with insecure patterns – resistant or avoidant – are also attached to their parents, and just as strongly as 'secure' infants. The insecure pattern of attachment is mostly an adaptive behaviour (due to the child's or the primary carer's temperament or behaviour) for obtaining the required response from their carers, and can also be a transient response following periods of separation from their carers. The prevalence of different attachment patterns varies with social risk factors. Higher prevalence of insecure and disorganised attachment patterns is seen in children with higher risk factors (Cyr *et al*. 2010). Current research indicates that a persistently poor parent–child relationship is largely responsible for long-term difficulties in social relationships rather than the early insecure attachment pattern per se (Grossman *et al*. 2005).

Secure: Infants use mothers as a secure base for exploration, protest when the caregiver leaves, are happy to see the caregiver return and recover quickly from any distress. In low-risk samples 65 per cent of children show this pattern.

Insecure:
■ *Avoidant*: 20 per cent of infants seem indifferent towards their caregiver and may even avoid the caregiver. When they get upset they are comforted as easily by a stranger as by a parent.

■ *Resistant or ambivalent*: 10 per cent of infants or young children are clingy, show poor exploratory behaviour, and get very upset when the caregiver leaves. They are not easily comforted and simultaneously seek comfort but also resist efforts by the caregivers to comfort them. The caregiver is often inconsistent in their availability to the child.

Disorganised/disoriented:
15 per cent of infants or young children have no consistent way of showing attachment to their caregiver or coping with the situation of being left alone with a stranger. Their behaviour is often confused or even contradictory, such as approaching the caregiver but being fearful (Main and Soloman 1986).

Disorganised attachment is not an indicator of insecurity, but of the child's disorganised thinking and behaviour and most likely results from a combination of child- and parent-related factors. It is more commonly seen in children with a history of maltreatment and abuse (up to 65 per cent) as compared to other children in the community (15 per cent). Infants with disorganised attachment patterns are at a higher risk of developing a range of emotional-behavioural difficulties and disorders in later life.

COMPANION @ WEBSITE

attachment disorders

Factors that contribute to insecure attachment relationships

Stressful events are part of life for most children and, in the context of good attachment relationships, do not result in lasting insecurity. Children's sense of insecurity is increased in the following situations (Kobak and Madsen 2008):

- Disrupted communications and a lack of responsiveness from carers (e.g. some parents with mental health problems).

- Carer leaving in an angry way with uncertainty of whereabouts.

- Parents threatening to leave or to send the child away.

- Parental threats of self-harm often occurring in the context of hostile and conflictual relationships.

- The child witnessing domestic violence.

- Parental conflicts often preceding separation, creating a fear that a parent may leave and never return.

Supporting secure attachments

Maintaining good open communication even in stressful situations can increase the confidence in the child about parental availability. Parental discipline accompanied with communication of clear expectations and rules rather than hostile and harsh remarks allows the child to appraise the situation better and adjust his/her behaviour accordingly (Kobak and Madsen 2008). Perceptive parents recognise the connection between a child's angry and oppositional behaviour and his/her fears about parental availability and maintain open communication to address these fears. Parents can maintain an attachment relationship with the child, even if separation is unavoidable, by engaging in a joint ongoing project (e.g. putting together a large complex puzzle or building a model or sewing an item of clothing or an outdoor activity) which would take several days and can be returned to until the child's insecure behaviour settles. Such activities can provide a focus for ongoing interaction and discussion between the parent and the child (Main *et al.* 2011).

TEMPERAMENT

Parents and carers are often aware of the differences in the style of how children usually approach and respond to situations. These differences in children's social approach, emotional reactions, attention and motor activity seem to have some consistency across situations and time. For example, some infants are more easily upset while others are easy-going; some appear more fearful or inhibited while others seem a bit too eager to join in and wade through obstacles.

Rothbart (2011) has described four main temperamental tendencies or traits (see Box 12). These traits are biologically based, i.e. there is a genetic predisposition for them, but they are shaped by parenting and caregiving processes. They become noticeable during early development and have a moderate degree of continuity over time. However, this is not to say that children's behaviour becomes predetermined because of their temperament; even the same child behaves differently in different situations and at different times because of their learning, cognitive ability, motivation and social constraints.

BOX 12 The structure of temperament in childhood (Rothbart 2011)

Four main temperament types have emerged from studies:

1. Surgency: it combines a disposition towards the positive emotions, rapid approach to potential rewards and a high activity level. These features can be observed as early as 2–3 months in smiling/laughter, vocal reactivity and activity.

2. Negative emotionality: fear and anger/frustration:

   ■ Fear: by 10 months some infants show fear/inhibition/distress on exposure to novel high-intensity toys. It predicts later fear and shyness to strangers when children are 7 years old. It protects children from approaching potentially harmful situations.

   ■ Anger/frustration: this is apparent from 2–3 months and occurs when a child's aims or expectations are denied and expresses as hitting, pushing and banging. It is an assertive form of negative emotionality and relates with higher aggression in late childhood.

3. Effortful control: this includes voluntary attentional focusing, inhibiting actions for immediate rewards and better planning abilities. This appears from 18–24 months and undergoes rapid development up to 7 years of age. With effortful control children choose to approach situations in a certain way.

4. Affiliation: it is a recent consideration in the description of temperament in children and relates to a behavioural style that expresses affectionate connection with others. It is a general disposition to experiencing pleasure in social behaviour.

Depending on their temperament children show differential sensitivity to punishments and rewards.

Children's temperament can be an important influence on parent–child relationship, family functioning, peer relationships and the child's participation in learning activities (Sanson *et al.* 2004).

An understanding of the child's temperament can help improve parents' awareness of a source of common difficulties and how a given style of parenting may be more or less helpful for their child. For example, children high in fear or inhibition respond better to a firm but gentle setting of boundaries and discipline rather than to permissive parenting. More active and positive children do better when parents are responsive to their need for stimulation and exploration (Putnam *et al.* 2002).

THE DEVELOPMENT OF SELF

The way children view themselves appears to influence the overall feelings of well-being and competence. The sense of self emerges early in infancy and is an ongoing and complex process.

Becoming self-aware

Early precursors of self-awareness are seen in infants' social interest in others. By 4 months of age, infants begin to show social interest in others and initiate vocal and gestural interactions with others. From 7 to 9 months they search visually for their parents and from 9 to 12 months establish *joint attention* with others to share their interests, indicating that they have a sense of separation from others. By the middle of the second year they recognise that a mirror image is a self-reflection, not a playmate, and on noticing a mark on their face they try to remove it from their face and not from the mirror. By the age of 2 years, children begin to insist on doing things for themselves and begin to use personal pronouns, e.g. me and mine, pick themselves out from pictures, show emotions of embarrassment and shame, and assert themselves through temper tantrums. Parents help the development of social self-assertion by setting limits and giving approval and praise for their actions. At about the same time, they also have a better sense of their physical self and make fewer 'scale-errors' – e.g. trying to sit in a toy chair.

Developing a categorical sense of self (self-definition)

As children develop language they begin to describe themselves on the basis of their distinct attributes and behaviour. From 2 years of age they tell their name and over the next few months begin to describe their gender (boy or girl) and whether they are big or little. From about 3 years, children describe their likings – they declare what they want to be in a role-play activity 'daddy, mummy or teacher' and what they are good at, e.g. 'running'. They also become aware of others' intentions and desires and take these into account in their actions. From the age of about 4 years they become aware that others' interpretation of situations may be different from their own. By the age of 5–6 years children distinguish between the 'inner', private self and the 'outer' presenting self – the way they ought to present themselves to others – and begin to hide their feelings from others (Rothbart 2011).

Parents contribute to the child's developing self-image by giving praise, positive or negative descriptions of their behaviour and by reminding them of their successes or failures. This influences children's perceptions of themselves, which, in turn, plays a role in how they respond to other task difficulties in the future. Some children, when faced with a difficulty or failure, blame themselves and stop trying whilst others persevere. Children who are supported in verbalising, analysing and describing their negative beliefs about themselves, given opportunities to succeed and praised for achieving success, have fewer problem behaviours and a better sense of self-esteem.

Supporting self-esteem

Further reading

Cassidy, J. and Shaver, P. R. (eds) (2008) *Handbook of Attachment*, 2nd edn. New York: The Guilford Press.

Rothbart, M. K. (2011) *Becoming Who We Are: Temperament and Personality in Development*. New York: The Guilford Press.

Zenah, C. H., Berlin, L. J. and Boris, N. W. (2011) 'Practitioner Review: Clinical Applications of Attachment Theory and Research for Infants and Young Children', *Journal of Child Psychology and Psychiatry* 52 (8): 819–33.

Vision and hearing

Vision and hearing are the essential sensory modalities for the development of non-verbal and verbal skills. Impairments in these sensory modalities are relatively common and, when significant, can permanently affect a child's development.

VISION

Functional vision is relatively poor at birth, but improves quickly over the next few weeks and months, reaching near adult levels by 6–8 months of age. As a major sensory modality, improving vision enables a child to perceive and interact with the social and physical world. Awareness of this changing visual behaviour (Table 12) is useful for eliciting information from parents and making observations.

Table 12 Development of observable visual behaviour.

Response to light	Blinks to flash and turns to diffuse light	Newborn
Visual awareness and interest	Shows special interest in human face and stares at objects held close to face	First month
Visual following	Follows faces and objects held near face Watches own hands Watches adult at 1.5 metres	6–8 weeks 3 months 4 months
Sharp visual fixation	Fixates 1-inch cube at 30 centimetres Fixates 1.5 mm (100s and 1000s) at 30 centimetres	5 months 9 months[1]
Visual acuity[2]	Can match picture of reducing sizes, e.g. Kay picture test Can match letters, e.g. Sonksen Silver acuity test[3]	2–2½ years 3½–4 years

[1] Functional vision, including depth perception, is at the near adult level by 8–9 months.
[2] *Visual acuity*, which requires more refined visual discrimination ability, reaches adult levels by the age of 4 years.
[3] The tests of visual acuity are best done by an orthoptist.

Poor visual behaviour, the presence of a *squint* or abnormal eye movements can be presenting features of a rare but serious eye condition or systemic disorders such as a cataract, glaucoma and retinoblastoma, which are sight- or life-threatening and are treatable.

Red-flag signs of possible vision problems

■ Not looking at carer's face or a bright object held close (about 30 centimetres) to the face by 6 weeks.

■ Not responding to carer's expressions or not giving eye contact by 8 weeks.

■ Not showing interest in or not reaching to pick up small toys or objects by 5 months.

■ Absence of sharp visual fixation to 1–1.5 mm colourful objects (e.g. small sweets, 'hundreds and thousands') after 9 months.

■ Looking at objects too closely after 12 months.

■ Erratic eye movements (any age).

■ Eyes that cross, turn in or out, move independently (any age).

■ Turning or tilting head to use only one eye to look at things (any age).

■ Poking or rubbing of eyes (any age).

HEARING

Due to the impact of impaired hearing on the development of language, reading and behavioural regulation, proactive enquiry of concerns, risk factors and tests of hearing are part of the children's surveillance programme. Awareness of the observable hearing behaviour and risk factors (Box 13) forms the basis for proactive inquiry from parents and for a referral to local audiology services.

At birth, infants show a preference for their mother's speech. This is likely to be based on the developing ability to hear from about 20 weeks of gestation, becoming well established by about 35 weeks of gestation (Hepper and Shahidullah 1994). Newborns are able to discriminate the general direction of a sound (left or right, far or near), but orienting towards more subtle variations in location improves over the next six months. Infants can discriminate vowels after birth; by 2–3 months they can discriminate the fine differences between phonemes such as /da/, /ba/ and /pa/, and by 6 months their speech discrimination is well refined. In some aspects infants' speech discrimination is better than that of adults. Before 6 months infants can discriminate speech sounds in their own and in other languages. However, by 10–12 months infants' speech perception becomes more like adults', with reduced perception of sounds in other languages. Children growing up with exposure to more than one language maintain their ability for discrimination of sounds in the languages used.

Tests for hearing, behavioural or physiological, are best conducted by audiology services. Subjective impressions or poorly done behavioural tests of hearing, which require proper training and suitable testing environment, can cause delay in identification of hearing impairment.

BOX 13 Risk factors for congenital or acquired hearing loss

■ Family history of sensorineuronal hearing loss.

■ History of maternal infection during pregnancy, e.g. toxoplasmosis, rubella, herpes, cytomegalovirus and syphilis.

■ Ear and other craniofacial anomalies.

■ Hyperbilirubinimia at levels requiring exchange transfusion.

■ Birthweight less than 1500 grams.

■ Genetic syndromes known to include Sensory Neuronal Hearing Loss (SNHL), e.g. Down's Syndrome, Waardenburg Syndrome.

■ Childhood disease associated with SNHL, e.g. meningitis, mumps, measles.

■ Ototoxic medication, e.g. Gentamicin.

■ Recurrent or persistent middle ear effusion ('glue ear') for at least three months.

---

domains of developmental progress

- Head trauma with fracture of temporal bone.

- *Neurodegenerative disease*, e.g. Hunter's syndrome, or demyelinating disease, e.g. Friedrich's ataxia, Charcot-Marie-Tooth syndrome.

- Lack of awareness to the usual environmental sounds, e.g. TV, sirens, 'pings' of the microwave/telephone etc., doorbell.

- Not responding when called.

- Listening to TV/radio/music at loud volume.

- Inattentiveness.

- Being unsettled at nursery/school.

- Stopping to vocalise after early babbling or other speech and language problems or talking too loudly.

- Discharge from ears, ear infections.

Red-flag signs of possible hearing problems

It may be difficult to differentiate between impaired hearing and inattention to speech observed in social communication disorder and an audiological assessment should be arranged in these situations.

Practitioners should clarify and confirm any concerns from parents and have a low threshold for making a referral to an audiologist or orthoptist/ophthalmologist, as per the local service policy or availability. Children with poor hearing or vision may also require developmental guidance, and early educational advice by specialist teachers, requiring a referral to the local services.

WHAT TO DO IF THERE IS A CONCERN REGARDING VISION OR HEARING

Glossary

The words from this Glossary can be found either in the text, the companion website and/or the accompanying videos.

Agency: the idea that people make events happen through their internal motivation.

Attention: concentration and focusing of mental resources.

Audiometry: the testing of a person's ability to hear various sound frequencies. The test is performed with an audiometer.

Babble: infants' vocalisation of reduplicated sequences of consonant–vowel syllables which function as the building blocks of words.

Cephalocaudal pattern: muscle tone and strength develop first in the muscles supporting the head and gradually spread towards feet.

Cognition: psychological processes that lead to 'knowing', e.g. attending, remembering, symbolising, representing.

Contexts: unique combinations of personal and environmental circumstances that can result in different paths of development, e.g. historical, family, economic and social factors.

Cooperative play: play that involves social interaction in a group, with a sense of organised activity.

Definition-by-use: child, when given an object, plays with it in an appropriate way, e.g. spoon in the mouth, brush on hair.

Developmentally vulnerable: susceptibility to poor developmental outcomes due to genetic, physical, cognitive or temperamental factors.

Developmental milestones: a developmental ability that is achieved by most children at a certain age.

Domain-specific: related to a specific domain of development, e.g. language or fine motor.

Dynamic: a continuous and systemic process of change and development.

Echolalia: repeating what someone says.

Executive functions: the monitoring and self-regulation of thought and action, to plan behaviour and to inhibit inappropriate responses.

Facilitative guidance: general guidance to parents and carers to promote the child's development.

False belief: an understanding that others may have beliefs that do not reflect current reality.

Functional difficulties: reported difficulties in day-to-day activities, e.g. playing, communicating, learning or socialising.

Gait: a person's manner of walking.

Genetic expression: the process by which information from a gene is used in the synthesis of a functional gene product, e.g. proteins, hormones and enzymes.

Global developmental delay: impairment of developmental progress in two or more domains (involving aspects of both verbal and non-verbal development).

Guttural sounds: sounds produced at the back of the mouth, usually vowels and usually of a harsh quality.

Hypothalamic Pituitary Adrenal (HPA) axis: the HPA axis refers to the hypothalamic-pituitary-adrenocortical axis. It is the internal neuroendocrine system that responds to stress and results in production of corticosteroid hormones that affect the brain, the cardiovascular system, and other systems in getting the body ready for what is known as the 'fight or flight' mechanism.

Hypo/hypertonia: decreased/increased muscle tone.

Impulsivity: acting before thinking; erratic and poorly controlled behaviour.

Intrinsic reinforcements: inner satisfaction and enjoyment from completing a task as opposed to external rewards.

Jargon: 'conversational babbling' or pre-linguistic vocalisations of young children that consist of several strings of consonants and vowels and may sound like connected speech, even though they are not true words. Jargon may have stress and the intonation patterns of connected speech.

Joint attention: is the shared focus of two individuals on an object. It is achieved when one individual alerts another to an object by means of eye-gazing, pointing or other verbal or non-verbal indications.

Make-believe play: a type of play in which children act out everyday and imaginary activities.

Metacognition: being aware of one's own thought processes including identifying problems, formulating solutions to solve problems, and so forth.

Micro/macrocephaly: a head circumference (HC) more than two standard deviation below/above the mean for age and gender.

Muscle tone: the continuous and passive partial contraction of the muscles, or the muscle's resistance to passive stretch during resting state.

Neonate: infant within age range of birth to 4 weeks.

Neurodegenerative disease: diseases resulting in the progressive loss of structure or function of neurons.

Neurotransmitters: chemicals released by neurons that cross the synapse to send messages to other neurons.

Norms/normative: when and how most children achieve a developmental ability.

Nystagmus: rapid involuntary movements of the eyes.

Object manipulation: hand-guided motor actions such as coordinated looking, rotating, transferring and fingering that facilitate infants' understanding of objects and about events involving objects.

Object permanence/Permanence of object: the understanding that objects continue to exist when they are out of sight.

Operant conditioning: a method of learning that occurs through rewards and punishments for behaviour. Through these rewards and punishments, an association is made between behaviour and a consequence for that behaviour.

Perceptual feedback: Perception is influenced by expectation or belief; feedback from experience confirms or modifies such expectations or beliefs.

Perinatal period: the time period starting at 22 completed weeks of gestation and lasting for seven days after birth.

Plasticity: the potential for relative systematic change in human development across the lifespan.

Popliteal angle: the angle between thigh and calf (femur and tibia) measured in supine position with the hip flexed 90° and the knee extended.

Premature (preterm): infant born before 37 weeks of gestation.

Pretend play: play involving acting out ideas and emotions. Children act out actions and stories that contain different perspectives and ideas.

Proprioception: the ability to sense the position, location, orientation and movement of the body and its parts.

Red flag: outlines a range of functional indicators or domains commonly used to monitor healthy child development, as well as potential problem areas for child development. It is intended to assist in the determination of when and where to refer for additional advice, formal assessment and/or treatment.

Red reflex: refers to the reddish-orange reflection of light from the eye's retina that is observed when using an ophthalmoscope from approximately 30 centimetres/1 foot.

Scaffolding: a process by which adults support and guide children's learning, enabling children to reach the next level of ability, beyond their own personal capability at that time. The term was coined by Bruner, building on Vygotsky's work.

Sensitive period: a time that is optimal for certain developmental capacities to emerge and in which the individual is especially responsive to environmental influences.

Sensitive-responsive parenting: parenting that involves responding promptly, consistently, and appropriately to infants and holding them tenderly and carefully.

Social referencing: using feedback from others to determine how to respond.

Social smile: the smile evoked by the stimulus of the human face. First appears between 6 and 10 weeks.

Squint: a deviation in the direction of the gaze of one eye.

Stranger wariness: expression of fear in response to unfamiliar adults, which appears in many babies in the second half of the first year.

Theory of Mind: the ability to accredit mental states to self and others.

Transactional process: a mutually interactive process in which children and the environment simultaneously influence each other, producing developmental change in both over time.

Visual acuity: sharpness of vision, which may be measured by the ability to discern letters or numbers at a given distance according to a fixed standard.

Walking base: describes how close (narrow base) or far apart (wide base) both legs are kept while walking.

Working memory: the memory system that temporarily keeps in information just received.

References

Adolph, K. E. and Berger, S. E. (2006) 'Motor Development', in D. Kuhn and R. S. Siegler (eds), *Handbook of Child Psychology, Vol. 2: Cognition, Perception, and Language*, 6th edn. New York: Wiley, pp. 161–213.

Adolph, K. E. and Berger, S. E. (2011) 'Physical and Motor Development', in M. H. Bornstein and M. E. Lamb (eds), *Cognitive Development: An Advanced Textbook*. New York: Psychology Press, pp. 257–318.

Adolph, K. E., Vereijken, B. and Denny, M. A. (1998) 'Learning to Crawl', *Child Development* 69 (5): 1299–312.

Adolph, K. E., Vereijken, B. and Shrout, P. E. (2003) 'What Changes in Infant Walking and Why', *Child Development* 74 (2): 475–97.

Ainsworth, M. D. S., Bleha, M., Waters, S. E. and Wall, S. (1978) *Patterns of Attachment: A Psychological Study of the Strange Situation*. Hillsdale, NJ: Erlbaum.

Amiel-Tison, C. and Grenier, A. (1986) *Neurological Assessment during the First Year of Life*. Oxford: Oxford University Press.

Baird, G., Charman, T., Baron-Cohen, S., Cox, A., Swettenham, J., Wheelwright, S. and Drew, A. (2000) 'A Screening Instrument for Autism at 18 Months of Age: A 6-Year Follow-Up Study', *Journal of the American Academy of Child and Adolescent Psychiatry* 39 (6): 694–702.

Bayley, N. (1969) *Bayley Scales of Infant Development*. New York: Psychological Corporation.

Belsky, J. and Most, R. K. (1981) 'From Exploration to Play', *Developmental Psychology* 17: 630–9.

Berger, A., Kofman, O., Livneh, U. and Henik, A. (2007) 'Multidisciplinary Perspective on Attention and the Development of Self-regulation', *Progress in Neurobiology* 82: 256–86.

Brazelton, T. B. and Nugent, J. K. (1995) *The Neonatal Behavioral Assessment Scale*. Cambridge: MacKeith Press.

Bruner, J. (1983) *Child's Talk: Learning to Use Language*. New York: W. W. Norton.

Cohen, D. (2006) *The Development of Play*, 3rd edn. Hove: Routledge.

Cooper, J., Moodley, M. and Reynell, J. (1978) *Helping Language Development: A Developmental Programme for Children with Early Learning Handicaps*. London: Edward Arnold.

Curry, N. E. and Arnaud, S. E. (1984) 'Play in Preschool Settings', in T. Yawkey and A. Pellegrini (eds), *Child's Play, Developmental and Applied*. London: Lawrence Erlbaum, pp. 53–67.

Cyr, C., Euser, E. M., Bakermans-Kranenburg, M. J. and van Ijzendoorn, M. H. (2010) 'Attachment Security and Disorganization in Maltreating and High-risk Families: A Series of Metaanalyses', *Development and Psychopathology* 22: 87–108.

Fenson, L., Dale, P. S., Reznick, J. S., Thal, D., Bates, E., Hartung, J. P., Pethick, S. and Reilly, J. S. (1993) *MacArthur Communicative Development Inventory: User's Guide and Technical Manual*. Baltimore, MD: Paul H. Brookes.

Fenson, L., Dale, P. S., Reznick, J. S., Bates, E., Thal, J. S., Pethick, S. J., Tomasello, M., Mervis, C. B. and Stiles, J. (1994) 'Variability in Early Communicative Development', *Monographs of the Society for Research in Child Development* 59 (5): i+iii–v, 1–185.

Frankenburg, W. K., Dodds, J. B., Fandal, A. W., Kazuk, E. and Cohrs, M. (1975) *The Denver Developmental Screening Test*. Denver, CO: University of Colorado Medical Center.

Galluhe, D. I. and Ozmum, J. C. (2006) *Understanding Motor Development*, 6th edn. New York: McGraw-Hill.

Garon, N., Bryson, S. E. and Smith, I. M. (2008) 'Executive Function in Preschoolers: A Review Using an Integrative Framework', *Psychological Bulletin* 134 (1): 31–60.

Grossman, K. E., Grossman, K. and Waters, E. (eds) (2005) *Attachment from Infancy to Adulthood*. New York: The Guilford Press.

Hepper, P. G. and Shahidullah, B. S. (1994) 'Development of Fetal Hearing', *Archives of Disease in Childhood* 71: F81–F87.

Holm, A., Stow, C. and Dodd, B. (2005) 'Bilingual Children with Phonological Disorders: Identification and Intervention', in B. Dodd (ed.), *Differential Diagnosis and Treatment of Children with Speech Disorder*, 2nd edn. London: Whurr, pp. 275–88.

I CAN (2006) *The Cost to the Nation of Children's Poor Communication*. London: I CAN.

Keller, H. (2003). 'Socialization for Competence: Cultural Models for Infancy', *Human Development* 46: 288–311.

Kobak, R. and Madsen, S. (2008) 'Disruptions in Attachment Bonds: Implications for Theory, Research, and Clinical Intervention', in J. Cassidy and P. R. Shaver (eds), *Handbook of Attachment: Theory, Research, and Clinical Applications*, 2nd edn. New York: Guilford Press, pp. 23–47.

Kopp, C. B. (1982) 'Antecedents of Self-regulation: A Developmental Perspective', *Developmental Psychology* 18 (2): 199–214.

Kopp, C. B. and Wyer, N. (1994) 'Self-regulation in Normal and Atypical Development', in D. Cicchetti and S. L. Toth (eds), *Rochester Symposium on Developmental Psychopathology, Vol. 5: Disorders and Dysfunctions of the Self*. New York: University of Rochester Press, pp. 31–56..

Locke, A., Ginsborg, J. and Peers, I. (2002) 'Development and Disadvantage: Implications for the Early Years and Beyond', *International Journal of Language and Communication Disorders* 37 (1): 3–16.

Lockman, J. J. (2005) 'Tool Use from a Perception–Action Perspective: Developmental and Evolutionary Considerations', in V. Roux and B. Bril (eds), *Stone Knapping: The Necessary Conditions for a Uniquely Hominid Behaviour*. London: Cambridge University Press, pp. 319–30.

McCune-Nicolich, L. (1981) 'Towards Symbolic Functioning', *Child Development* 52: 785–97.

Main, M. and Soloman, J. (1986) 'Discovery of an Insecure Disorganized/ Disorientated Attachment Pattern: Procedures, Findings and Implications for the Classification of Behaviour', in T. B. Brazelton and M. Yogman (eds), *Affective Development in Infancy*. Norwood, NJ: Ablex, pp. 95–124.

Main, M., Hesse, E. and Hesse, S. (2011) 'Attachment Theory and Research: Overview with Suggested Applications to Child Custody', *Family Court Review* 49 (3): 426–3.

Marvin, R. S. and Britner, P. A. (2008) 'Normative Development: The Ontogeny of Attachment', in J. Cassidy and P. R. Shaver (eds), *Handbook of Attachment*, 2nd edn. New York: The Guilford Press, pp. 269–94.

Milani-Comparetti, A. and Gidoni, E. A. (1967) 'Routine Developmental Examination in Normal and Retarded Children', *Developmental Medicine and Child Neurology* 9 (9): 631–8.

Nelson, K. (2007) *Young Minds in Social World: Experience, Meaning and Memory*. Cambridge, MA: Harvard University Press.

Omkloo, H. (2007) 'Fitting Objects into Holes: On the Development of Spatial Cognition Skills', *Acta Universitatis Upsaliensis*. Digital Comprehensive Summaries of Uppsala Dissertations from the Faculty of Social Sciences, 34, 84 pp., Uppsala.

Pellegrini, A. D. (2009) *The Role of Play in Human Development*. Oxford: Oxford University Press.

Piek, J. P. (2006) *Infant Motor Development*. Champaign, IL: Human Kinetics.

Prechtl, H. F. R. (1977) *The Neurological Examination of the Fullterm Newborn Infant*, 2nd edn. Clinics in Developmental Medicine 63. London: MacKeith Press.

Putnam, S. P., Sanson, A. and Rothbart, M. K. (2002) 'Child Temperament and Parenting', in M. H. Bornstein (ed.), *Handbook of Parenting*, 2nd edn, *Vol. 1: Children and Parenting*. Hillsdale, NJ: Lawrence Erlbaum Associates, pp. 255–78.

RCSLT (2003) *Core Guidelines*. London: RCSLT.

Robson, P. (1984) 'Prewalking Locomotor Movements and Their Use in Predicting Standing and Walking', *Child Care Health and Development* 10 (5): 317–30.

Rothbart, M. K. (2011) *Becoming Who We Are: Temperament and Personality in Development*. New York: The Guilford Press.

Ruff, H. A. and Rothbart, M. K. (1996) *Attention in Early Development*. New York: Oxford University Press.

Sanson, A., Hemphill, S. A. and Smart, D. (2004) 'Connections between Temperament and Social Development: A Review', *Social Development* 13 (1): 142–70.

Stiles, J. and Stern, C. (2001) 'Developmental Change in Spatial Cognitive Processing: Complexity Effects and Block Construction Performance in Preschool Children', *Journal of Cognition and Development* 2 (2): 157–87.

Stiles-Davis, J. (1988) 'Developmental Change in Young Children's Spatial Grouping Activity', *Developmental Psychology* 24: 522–31.

Tamis-LeMonda, C. S. and Adolph, K. E. (2005) 'Social Cognition in Infant Motor Action', in B. Homer and C. S. Tamis-LeMonda (eds), *The Development of Social Cognition and Communication*. Mahwah, NJ: Erlbaum, pp. 145–64.

Thelen, E. (1995) 'Motor Development: A New Synthesis', *American Psychologist* 50 (2): 79–95.

Thompson, R. A. (2008) 'Early Attachment and Later Development: Familiar Questions and New Answers', in J. Cassidy and P. R. Shaver (eds), *Handbook of Attachment*, 2nd edn. New York: The Guilford Press, pp. 348–65.

Thompson, R. A., Virmani, E. A., Waters, S. F., Raikes, H. A. and Meyer, S. (2013) 'The Development of Emotional Self-regulation: The Whole and the Sum of Parts', in K. C. Barrett, N. A. Fox, G. A. Morgan, D. A. Fidler and L. A. Daunhauer (eds), *Handbook of Self-regulatory Processes*. New York: Psychology Press, pp. 5–26.

Trevarthen, C. and Aitken, K. J. (2001) 'Infant Intersubjectivity: Research, Theory, and Clinical Applications', *Journal of Child Psychology and Psychiatry* 42 (1): 3–48.

Zenah, C. H., Berlin, L. J. and Boris, N. W. (2011) 'Practitioner Review: Clinical Applications of Attachment Theory and Research for Infants and Young Children', *Journal of Child Psychology and Psychiatry* 52 (8): 819–33.